Doctors, Patients, and Placebos

DOCTORS, PATIENTS, AND PLACEBOS

Howard M. Spiro, M.D.

YALE UNIVERSITY PRESS
New Haven and London

Designed by Susan P. Fillion and set in Baskerville
text and Helvetica display type by Eastern Graphics.
Printed in the United States of America by Halliday
Lithograph, West Hanover, Mass.

Library of Congress Cataloging-in-Publication Data

Spiro, Howard M. (Howard Marget), 1924–
    Doctors, patients, and placebos.

    Includes index.
    1. Medicine and psychology. 2. Placebo (Medicine)
3. Physician and patient. 4. Sick—Psychology.
I. Title. [DNLM: 1. Drug Therapy—psychology.
2. Physician-Patient Relations. WB 330 S759d]
R726.5.S64   1986   615.5'8'019   86-5593
ISBN 0-300-03303-6 (alk. paper)

*The paper in this book meets the guidelines for permanence
and durability of the Committee on Production Guidelines
for Book Longevity of the Council on Library Resources.*

10 9 8 7 6 5 4 3 2 1

Contents

To my patients, who have taught me so much,
in sickness and in health

Acknowledgments

To acknowledge fully my indebtedness for the ideas in this book would be to list my teachers, my patients, and many colleagues at Yale University. I record then only a special indebtedness to the Center for Advanced Studies in Behavioral Sciences at Stanford, California, where I was a Fellow for the academic year 1982–83. There I found a relaxed and nondirective collegiality which encouraged me to sit back, look around, and contemplate where I had been and where I should go. Gardner Lindzey, its jolly and wise Director, advised me to come without a plan, forecasting that the book I did not write would be better than the book I did write (I hope he is wrong). The Center gave me the chance to read in many different areas without conscious direction. As I did so, I became aware of how much of my professional practice had been circling around problems of pain, and the idea of this book gradually took shape.

In 1955, when I came to New Haven, there were five gastroenterologists in Connecticut, a state then with slightly less than three million people. In those days I saw mainly people with organic diseases, with cancer of the colon or stomach, colitis or pancreatitis, problems which called for a specific diagnostic approach and a relatively standard therapy. The three decades since have seen the population of Connecticut grow only slightly, to something over three million, but the number of gastroenterologists increase from 5 to about 185. Regardless of the improvement such inflation has brought to the welfare of the Connecticut public, the ubiquity of gastroenterologists has changed the kinds of patients who come to see me. People with readily recognizable diseases usually have no need of university physicians, and so many of my patients have complaints of pain for which their doctors cannot immediately find a source or origin and which find no reflection in myriad imaging studies. Pain and its relief have become central concerns in my outpatient consultative practice.

Equally important to my growing interest in pain has been the flowering of controlled clinical trials in gastroenterology, especially of peptic ulcer treatment. Such trials have underlined how readily ulcer pain disappears, as quickly relieved by a placebo as by an active drug.

At the Center I considered these phenomena, began to wonder how placebos worked, and from my reading and contemplation gradually put together the background for some reflections upon placebos and pain relief. While I have tried to review the available medical English-language literature on the general placebo phenomenon, I have not studied the psychiatric literature in any depth, nor have I made any attempt to evaluate specific placebo-controlled trials. Rather, I have looked at the general phenomenon of the placebo effect and what it suggests about clinical practice. I have tried to separate truth from hope. Thinking about the placebo led me to think also about medical practice, physician-patient relationships, and many other crucial issues which so challenge our time. I have had to comment on some of these matters, but only as they relate to placebo and pain relief.

All the fellows at the Center in 1982–83 had an influence on my thinking. I owe a special debt of gratitude to David Leary, whose study was next door to mine. A professor of psychology at the University of New Hampshire, David has a wide interest in the history of psychology and science; his eclectic but gentle stimulation led me to read far more generously than I might have on my own. Jim Fernandez, professor of anthropology at Princeton, called my attention to medical anthropology, a field of which I had been shamefully ignorant, and we had many useful chats. Richard Rorty, professor of philosophy at the University of Virginia, suggested a number of readings in pragmatic ways; I have read his books with benefit. The daily lunches at the Center were astonishingly instructive, but to these Fellows I owe the most. The travel circumscriptions of the Center kept me at Stanford. The Henry J. Kaiser Family Foundation supported me as a Senior Scholar during that year so very dear to me.

Harvey Mandell of Norwich, Connecticut, and I have had lunch together on Fridays for over thirty years. Together we have gained some weight but also some depth. Over that period our conversations and our collaborations have ranged widely. I am especially indebted to Harvey for his careful and generous review of the entire manuscript and his cheerful if sometimes quizzical puncture of my more gaseous balloons. He has helped to focus my thoughts and has sharpened my awareness of the challenges to the practicing physician in treating the pain patient.

Other colleagues have also been crucial in giving form to my reflections. At the Yale Law School Jay Katz and Robert Burt provided me with a five-year opportunity as part of the Law-Medicine Program to look at medicine from the outside. I have read their books, argued with them intermittently, so that my debt to them, and to the Commonwealth Fund support for that five years, is as much subliminal as conscious, the result of conversation as well as reading.

Marilyn and John Smith, professors of philosophy both, have been close friends and intellectual guides for many years, I owe an inexpressible debt of gratitude to them.

Robert Aronowitz as a senior medical student at Yale wrote his senior thesis on the psychosomatic hypothesis in inflammatory bowel disease at the time that I was preparing this book. We had many profitable discussions, and I owe much to his careful reading of the manuscript, which led to many changes. Jack Hughes, Director of the Outpatient Clinic at Yale-New Haven Hospital, offered valuable comments on the manuscript, and Paul Wolpe, a Ph.D. candidate in sociology at Yale, has also been among the more assiduous of my critics. I am beholden to them all.

My debt to Dr. Mack Lipkin, of North Carolina and of the world, is great indeed. I visited Mack in his gracious southern home to plunder his collection of materials on suggestion and the placebo, and to talk with him about my ideas. Dr. Carolyn Spiro-Winn, my psychiatrist-daughter, provided me with the materials on transference and counter-transference. Her skepticism has always sharpened my thoughts. James Pohlman, Esq., of Columbus, Ohio, provided me with the appropriate references on malpractice law and the placebo, for which I thank him here.

I have been lucky indeed to have the Yale University library available to me and luckier still in the reference librarians at the Medical School and at the University to help me in tracing down some attributions. Ed Tripp and Michael Joyce of the Yale University Press coaxed revision and pruning, for which the reader may be thankful. I am in their debt.

This manuscript has been in gestation on and off for three years. My secretary at the Center, Barbara Homestead, started out with this manuscript. Donna Dillon, Helen Lewis, Gale Iannone, and finally Caryl Foote, have all deserved more than mere reward in print because of their cheerful working and reworking of the manuscript. Caryl Foote has brought it to fruition, and I am especially grateful to her.

I should also call attention to writers who have been influential in my thinking about the placebo and who though listed over and over in my bibliography, deserve special thanks. They include George Engel, Jerome Frank, Howard Brody, Eric Cassell, and Norman Cousins.

Finally, Marian Spiro, my partner of thirty-five years, has made my life fuller; her questioning of my certainty has given me a richer and more critical point of view.

Throughout the book I have used the shorthand "he" for "she or he." I am grateful that medicine is now sex-blind, but my brain is too hard-wired for me to use the double pronoun of "him or her" or to use the female pronoun in every other chapter. Therefore, with admiration for women and with the understanding that "him" to me androgynously means man or woman, I have continued to use the male pronoun. If I offend in that, I am truly sorry.

1

Introduction

I have been using placebo therapy in what I thought was an honest way for a long time. Trying to relieve a patient with symptoms out of proportion to objective findings—particularly one complaining of pain the source of which I do not immediately recognize and which I suspect I will never be able to categorize, or someone with weakness and lassitude which does not fit into the category of depression—I have often suggested 1,000 micrograms of vitamin B-12 to be injected three times a week for a month. Customarily, I have told the patient something like this: "I'm going to have you get some B-12 injections. They have helped many other patients, but I cannot explain to you why they work and I cannot promise you they will work. I can simply say that many patients tell me they feel better and stronger after such a course of therapy." I have not kept numbers, but it is my impression that more people were helped than not, and I hope that no one has been harmed.

If I had been asked to say what had happened, I would have responded that even if the B-12 was a placebo, it lessened anxiety and gave hope and new strength because the patient expected that it would help him. I felt I had done my duty as a physician to relieve suffering, and that I had not deceived my patients. Imagine my surprise, then, to find that a philosopher and ethicist at the Center for Advanced Study in the Behavioral Sciences at Stanford, though he agreed that I knew what I was doing, suggested that in using a placebo I was deceiving my patients. Disturbed at this suggestion, I began to review what was known about placebos, how they work, their use and misuse, in order to respond to my philosopher friend and critic.

1

My primary medical education took place in the 1940s, and I was much entranced by the psychosomatic theories of those times. The common opinion of my teachers and models is probably expressed in a quotation from a 1943 book, *Psychosomatic Medicine*, now out of print and no longer even available in the Yale Medical Library. In that book Weiss and English said:

> The physician who prescribes placebos, in whatever form, is not consciously dishonest. He wants to help his patient. He knows his patient expects drug treatment. He is aware of the resistance of the patient to the idea that his symptoms are the result of emotional conflict. He (the doctor) has seen the beneficial effects of suggestion by placebos in other cases and hopes that the same thing will happen again. When he runs out of placebos the patient runs out on him.[1]

Norman Cousins, whose account I will review later, commented about his own illness:

> I have wondered, in fact, about the relative absence of attention given the placebo in contemporary medicine. . . . I was absolutely convinced, at the time I was deep in my illness, that intravenous doses of ascorbic acid could be beneficial—and they were. It is quite possible that this treatment—like everything else I did—was a demonstration of the placebo effect. If so, it would be just as important to probe into the nature of this psychosomatic phenomenon as to find out if ascorbic acid is useful in combatting a high sedimentation rate.[2]

Such comments fortified me in my examination of the placebo. Later I read Jay Katz's comment, "If placebos were to be acknowledged as effective in their own right, it would expose large gaps in medicine's and doctor's knowledge about underlying mechanisms of care and relief from suffering."[3] And that is what this book is about.

As I read, I became aware that studying the placebo was making me reexamine the emphasis on science that characterizes the present era, and the split between *care* and *cure*. The use of that word *care* has become a cliche, but it is no less real for being so hackneyed. Physicians in hospital training learn the virtues of *cure* but seldom of *care*, a catchphrase which says a great deal. They are taught that their goal is to detect and then cure diseases of all sorts, especially the acute ones

1. Weiss, E., and English, O. S., *Psychosomatic medicine*, Philadelphia: Saunders, 1943.

2. Cousins, N., Anatomy of an illness (as perceived by the patient). *NEJM*, 295: 1460–63, 1976.

3. Katz, J., *The silent world of doctor and patient*, New York: Free Press, 1984, p. 191.

they see in the hospital. Care is often ignored, though often complimented in texts and speeches at graduation exercises. Cure is directed at disease; care is directed at the patient who has an illness with complaints. Physicians try to cure acute diseases; we care for patients with chronic diseases which, by their nature, we only rarely cure. The placebo makes us focus on the patient.

This book is directed primarily to my colleagues in clinical medicine, who practice and who teach, and to medical students. My purposes in writing are several: (1) to suggest that the scientific approach to human disease and illness—the molecular model of medicine—is not sufficient by itself to answer all our patients' needs; (2) to reemphasize that disease differs from illness, that placebos help the illness component of the disease; (3) to suggest, as have many before me, that the patient's account is still important in suggesting what is wrong with him, what he is *suffering* from. The prized objectivity of the physician must yield somewhat to the patient's report. However objective he may wish to be, the physician has always to rely on the history, the story really, which is largely the patient's subjective report. I will comment later about interpreting images in the context of what the patient has to say. Relief of symptoms is important even when the physician is not sure what is wrong with the patient; and (4) most important to reassert the power of the physician in the healing act, the ability of one person to help another, and the power of community. The placebo reminds us that we are not alone; I doubt that one could give oneself a placebo, though the power of self-determination is great. The placebo celebrates healing and makes us physicians look at the whole person. In that respect, although I will underline some of my disagreements with the alternative medical movement, particularly the holistic acceptance of every anecdote as the equal of every other, we physicians need to recover a sense of the person in the patient.

Science, however, is still the base of medical practice, and on that foundation and from that perspective I will examine the placebo. Medical practice is stretched by the tensions between science and intuition; the lens of the placebo has helped me to focus on some of those strains in the practice of medicine, including cost restraints in a time of declining economy and increasing demand, the overuse of technology in the detection of disease, and the new ethical questions sprung from those new medical skills. There are others which we will encounter in this survey.

At Stanford I became aware of how important are the metaphors by which we live,[4] and how they define and limit what we physicians

4. Lakoff, G., and Johnson, M., Conceptual metaphor in everyday language, *J. Philosophy* 77:453–86, 1980.

do,[5] and what everyone else does too, for that matter. I have been convinced that an underlying problem, basic to everything else, is the model that physicians have developed for themselves: ever since the Enlightenment, physicians as a group have come to see themselves as physicists, not as poets. One of the reasons why we overtreat and over-study and cannot always talk with, or even listen to, our patients is that most of us are too busy looking at their organs and functions. The eye, as I will emphasize, rules the ear.

What had begun as a reexamination of my own use of the placebo expanded into some reflections on how physicians take care of patients. I fear that modern medical culture has somehow mistaken the means—science—for the end—caring for patients. In this short and admittedly personal account I can touch only a few topics. Still, I hope that my questions without answers will lead others, particularly medical students and young physicians, to examine where medical practice has been going and where changes are needed.

One reason for the overuse of technology comes from the emphasis during training that an answer can be found for everything if the physician will only look far and deep enough, and with enough instruments. Physicians are taught to find the cause of a symptom before treating it. To relieve symptoms, pain especially, without trying to ascertain its cause is nowadays denigrated as "bad" medicine; as an internist I recognize that automatically handing out pills without analyzing the patient's complaint will lead to trouble. But for many people symptom relief may be all that is needed; the patient is as important as his disease. To know this, of course, the physician must know his patient. That too is a commonplace, praised but not honored.

Modern physicians want hard data, hard copy, and the printout; they pay most attention to what has a proven relationship to disease and very much less to suffering. It makes little sense for physicians to adopt so precise an attitude toward tobacco and alcohol that they record in a medical history the pack-years of tobacco smoked and the grams of alcohol consumed, and yet pay so little attention to the personal, cultural, social, and other nonmeasurable features of the patient's life.

It was not always so. There was a time, most recently in the 1940s and 1950s, when a synthesis of social, psychic, and physical influences collectively known as psychosomatic medicine promised to provide a holistic view of patients.[6] At Yale in the 1920s the Institute of Human Relations, founded and fostered by Dean Milton Winternitz of the Medical School and President Rowland Angell of the University, tried

5. Fernandez, J., Persuasions and performances, *Daedalus* 110:39–60, 1971.
6. Weiss and English, *Psychosomatic medicine*.

to insert the social sciences and psychology into the medical curriculum to get physicians to consider more than the bodies of their patients.[7] They built a building, but that was all. The institute now houses a laboratory for genetics, and all that remains is the old name carved over the entrance to Yale Medical School. Molecular biology and genetic engineering hold sway, and few look back to the dreams of the 1920s.

The problem lies not only in the unconscious models which physicians have of sickness, but in their conscious concepts of the role of the physician. Over the past one hundred years the physician has seen himself in several different roles, as *practitioner* at the bedside, as *clinician* in a hospital, and as *scientist* in a laboratory. As Jewson points out,[8] the physician sitting at the bedside sees the patient as a person, looks at him as a whole person made up of a number of parts important only as they all work together. The clinician in the hospital concentrating on the disease, on the organic biological lesion, sees his patient as a case. Rather than listening to the patient to analyze his complaint, the hospital physician looks at the pathology, chemical or structural in nature. This stage, which the imaging revolution has renewed, accounts for some of the misunderstandings between patient and physician.

The third stage—laboratory medicine—which now dominates medical training turns the physician into a scientist studying the cell and its subcellular processes, tracing its DNA rather than listening to, or even looking at, the person who is the patient. Virchow, the great nineteenth-century pathologist, introduced the term "cellular pathology," emphasizing thereby that diseases begin in cells. The corresponding "cellular therapy," the treatment of those diseased cells, has eluded science until recently: the triumphs of genetic engineering suggest how close we are at present to cellular therapy. The introduction of the H2 blockers, to block the stimulation of the acid-secreting cells of the stomach, or even more impressively, the substituted benzimidazoles which work within the cell, suggest that drugs can now be seen at least as cellular in aim.[9] Recombinant DNA therapy, to supply missing or faulty functions to the cell, now so tantalizingly near, will prove to be that cellular therapy. Medical practice in the hospital swings between hospital medicine, with its focus on biologically de-

7. Viseltear, A. J., Milton C. Winternitz and the Yale Institute of Human Relations: A brief chapter in the history of social medicine, *Yale J. Biol. Med.* 57:869–89, 1984.

8. Jewson, N. D., The disappearance of the sick-man from medical cosmology, 1770–1870, *Sociology* 10:225–44, 1976.

9. Lauritsen, K., Rone, S. J., Bytzer, R., et al., Effect of omeprazole and cimetidine on duodenal ulcer, *NEJM* 312:958–61, 1985.

tectable organic structural lesions, and laboratory medicine that detects largely biochemical and immunological deviations.

At all three stages emphasis is placed on seeing, a problem to which I will return. The physician *sees* the patient, *sees* the subcellular processes. The function of the physician is to look, not so much to listen. So much do the metaphors of science and medicine come from seeing that the doctor's ear may atrophy from disuse.

The patient, however, has not changed; he just wants to get better. Most of us want to talk to our doctor, need some personal connection, and are understandably unenthusiastic about being a case. It is this divergent "cosmology," as Jewson puts it, which underlies much of the dissatisfaction with the medical community. Looking at the placebo, I will suggest, forces the physician to regard the patient as a whole person.

Of course, there are dangers in physicians assuming that someone who comes to them for relief of a specific complaint wants to be looked at as a whole person and that he is yearning to turn over his entire body for rehabilitation. Such enlarging of "medical space" is just what Illich warns against, "medicalizing" society.[10] Taking on too much responsibility is something that the physician has to guard against. Even worse, however, is looking at people only as collections of organs to be transplanted—or even substituted by—artificial devices.

Looking at placebo effects has led me to consider folk medicine, faith healing, and other arts slightly disreputable in medical circles. Looking at alternative medicine may provoke as much anxiety (or even anger) in other physicians as it has in me because it reminds us of the uncertain borders of our work; but a digression into anthropological studies of medical habits in other cultures may convince us that if patients come to physicians for comfort and relief of pain, we should analyze their problems as scientifically and logically as possible, without scorning unexplained and unscientific occurrences. Medical anthropology, which looks at how people in different cultures explain disease and how they go about seeking help, even how different ideas can cause disease (or at least define it), can widen the Western physician's views of what he is doing and make him more skeptical of some of his pursuits.

Let me emphasize once again how important it is to maintain a rational, logical, scientific approach in examining claims about the placebo and healing. Many enthusiastic but undocumented reports have been written without the skepticism which should attend clinical reports, quantitative or anecdotal. It is too easy, as too many advocates

10. Illich, I., *Medical nemesis*, London: Calder and Boyars, 1975, pp. 31–66.

of alternative medicine have done, to select out single observations, torn from their context, as stepping stones to unwarranted conclusions. In writing about the claim for acupuncture, for example, Skrabanek puts it well: "What is at issue is the complex problem of demarcation between science and quackery, between honest search for truth and unscrupulous exploitation of human suffering."[11]

Almost anything can be made to sound logical, and it is too easy, I have found, to become so entranced with rapturous reports of miracles or magic that one casts aside the scientific because it is so heavy, to take up the mystical because it requires no work. I hope that I have avoided such pitfalls by keeping foremost my scientific training as a physician and stressing the basis of reasoning that characterizes modern medicine. Scientific principles should be applied to evaluating even what seems to be unknown. We must remain committed to the scientific approach even in looking at the placebo and the plausible.

But there should be no forbidden questions.[12] Just because something seems irrational by the reigning paradigm is no reason not to examine it. But just because it opposes the majority view is no reason to hold it as valid! At a time of immunological miracles, of heart and gene transplants and the revelations of neurobiology, it is easy to direct all our energies toward the scientific frontier. In a time of war, to continue a medical metaphor, there is no leisure for doctors. Yet looking sideward or backward into the unknown shadows can be illuminating. Lying as it does at the border of the known and the unknown, the measurable and the unmeasurable, the rational and the mystical, the placebo has reminded me at a time when technology is triumphant that much of what we physicians do is still not grounded on reason and may never need to be. The placebo cuts through the patient-physician relationship to make us think about the role of the physician in the healing process. It expresses the tension between reason and intuition.

There is a long tradition in medicine going back to Hippocrates which looks with disdain on the purely anecdotal, but knowledge comes in classifying, analyzing, and testing hypotheses. Physicians need to ask *how* the placebo effect comes about and in what circumstances, instead of covering it with opprobrium because the phenomenon seems currently inaccessible to objective scientific assessment.

For example, until recent work on prostaglandins most physicians were unaware of how aspirin relieved pain. Yet they gave it, and took it themselves, because someone had "shown" that aspirin was effective, although they might not have been able to cite specific publica-

11. Skrabanek, P., Acupuncture and the age of unreason, *Lancet* 1:1169–71, 1984.
12. Turner, F., personal communication, 1984.

tions. Aspirin worked, and because it was sold as an analgesic, they had few questions about it. Now physicians have a more precise idea of how aspirin relieves pain, but that knowledge has not improved their practice. If they knew in the 1960s that aspirin raised the pain perception threshold, and in the 1970s that it worked by inhibiting prostaglandin synthetase, and in the 1980s that cyclooxygenase converts arachidonic acid from cell membranes to the prostaglandins, they understood more and more, but their practice remained unchanged. Clergymen contemplate the meaning of the rituals they lead, more than the congregants in the pews, but their prayers still sound the same. Physicians recommend the use of aspirin as a pain reliever, just as before. Physicians try to ground their practice, or are taught to anyway, in scientific medicine. If it turns out, as seems likely, that placebos relieve pain at least in part by stimulating endogenous endorphins, then we still must ask whether finding a mechanism for the subjective relief will justify the placebo—or whether, even if no current scientific validation of the mechanism is forthcoming, the observations of their benefit are any the less real.

To be sure, there is a big difference between observing, recording, and classifying stories of placebo relief and demonstrating or explaining their mechanisms. Observation is not explanation. I do not want to fall into the post hoc ergo propter hoc hole. But simply because we do not yet know how placebos work, need we discard them? If physicians had awaited an explanation of the benefits of penicillin on pneumonia, instead of relying on clinical experience, they would have waited many years. "Ah," but the reader may object, "doctors could take X-rays to see the pneumonia vanish. Penicillin cured pneumonia overnight. Placebos don't work in all patients!" Penicillin vanquished pneumococcal pneumonia, not viral pneumonia. Analyzing the circumstances in which placebos are effective is as necessary as categorizing the different kinds of pneumonia if we are to come up with rational observations. Finding a biologic explanation of how a placebo works is desirable, but will knowing that endorphin stimulation springs from faith make the question of deception redundant? Or make lying to patients physiologically respectable?

When we get to explanations, we must not be too beguiled by endorphin mechanisms, but recognize that anything which directs the attention of the patient away from his pain may be helpful. My daughter, now a psychiatrist, suggested to me many years ago that I could do without novocaine when I had a tooth filled if I thought "around my mouth." That is what happened! My attention was directed away from my tooth.

Finally, I hope that contemplation of the placebo and how—or whether—it works may help in the current reevaluation of the goals of medical practice, education, and diagnosis. College students study science to get into medical school; the goal of most medical students is to get a good residency to learn how to manage seriously ill patients in a hospital; and many residents aim at a subspecialty with enough tools to give them the reward of confidence that they are doing something worthwhile. After a decade or more of emphasis on disease the physician comes out into the world of the sick and worried-well and is ill prepared to deal with illness and pain except by technological pursuits. I hope that my review of the placebo as a link between doctor and patient will provide a little extra encouragement for people thinking about medical education. I know that exhortation alone almost never changes behavior, particularly when that behavior is reinforced by the rewards that the biomedical leaders can bestow. Still, I can hope to ask questions.

I have written this book for doctors and medical students, but I will be delighted if some laymen also read it for a glimpse of the uncertainties in medicine which even today too often lie veiled from them. Medical interest groups like the American Cancer Society have done enormous good, but they may have too zealously educated the public to believe that physicians have the answers to most diseases (or that with enough money and resources, research will provide them). As a result too many patients demand too many tests for too many minor complaints. Perhaps reading this book will help the lay public to tolerate medical uncertainty, even for themselves.

2
Definitions

There are four parts to the placebo transaction as it is usually enacted in modern medical practice: A *physician* gives what he believes to be an *inert material* to a *sick person*, with a complaint that may or may not originate in a biologically detectable disease, and after that, there is the *placebo effect*—the disease or the complaint improves. A distinction must be made between the placebo response *of* the person and the placebo effect *on* the disease. The patient may respond in some subjective way to the placebo, but that is different from the effect on a disease. Later we will scrutinize the evidence for cure of disease as contrasted with relief of symptom. For now let us accept that the physician, the placebo, the patient—and perhaps most important—the act of giving somehow combine to bring about the placebo effect. Our task is to examine the components. For simplicity I will limit the discussion to oral medication, though later I will consider to what degree operations, injections, and other maneuvers work as placebos.

It is important to begin by asking whether we are all referring to the same thing when we use the word *placebo*. The *Oxford English Dictionary* (1971) says that *placebo* was first used in matters ecclesiastical as the name given to Vespers in the Office for the Dead because the first antiphon began with the Latin *placebo* ("I shall please"). Verse 9 of Psalm 116 in the King James version of the Bible promises, "I will walk before the Lord in the land of the living." But we are assured that a translation error switched "I shall walk" to "I shall please."[1] (This is only the first of many errors in the history of the placebo!) The *OED* illustrates the early use of the word thus: "He earned a mis-

1. Shapiro, A. K., A contribution to a history of the placebo effect, *Behavioral Science* 5:109–35, 1960.

erable livelihood . . . by singing placebos and diriges." Even then the placebo was connected with money.

The word gradually attained a pejorative note and took on the allusion of "sycophant," "flatterer," and worse. Placebo was used in medical practice first as almost a synonym for any medicine and gradually became a synonym for an inert or harmless medicine calculated to please the patient. Shapiro, who has exhaustively analyzed the placebo problem and its history, records that placebo was first used in medical terms in 1785 to mean "commonplace method or medicine."[2] In 1811, so he tells us, the modern use of the term first came into being as "all medicine prescribed more to please the patient than for its therapeutic effectiveness."

Beecher, whose pioneering observations have formed the foundation of most subsequent observations, wrote in 1955 of its common purposes

> as a psychological instrument in the therapy of certain ailments arising out of mental illness, as a resource of the harassed doctor in dealing with a neurotic patient to determine the true effect of drugs apart from suggestion, in experimental work, as a device for eliminating bias not only on the part of the patients but also, when used as an unknown, of the observer, and, finally, as a tool of importance in the study of mechanisms of drug action.[3]

Today there are two major ways in which *placebo* is used in medical practice and writing, as *therapy* and as *substitute*. As we shall see, the placebo in practice and the placebo in research protocols are given in quite different spirit, so that it is important for us to keep their different roles clear. By the placebo as substitute I mean what the British call a dummy, an inactive drug used in controlled clinical trials. The first will engage most of our attention, but it is convenient to define the nontherapeutic use of placebo first.

PLACEBO AS DUMMY

The nontherapeutic use of an inactive agent called placebo should not be confused with the therapeutic placebo. Many physicians (I have been among them) participate in controlled clinical trials to test the benefit of a new drug on a disease. Duodenal ulcer offers a good example. In such a study a group of patients with dyspepsia and an

2. Shapiro, A. K., The placebo response, In *Modern perspectives in world psychiatry*, vol. 2, ed. J. G. Howells, Edinburgh: Oliver and Budy, 1971; and ibid.

3. Beecher, H. K., The powerful placebo, *JAMA* 159:1602–06, 1955.

ulcer crater seen at endoscopy receive a new drug for a defined period of time to find out whether the drug (1) relieves the pain or (2)
speeds the healing of the ulcer crater. But since duodenal ulcer craters tend to heal on their own, with almost any treatment (or indeed
on no treatment at all), it is necessary to compare the course of patients taking a new drug to that of others on no treatment or on a
proven drug believed to be less effective. For that reason another
group of patients are recruited to receive standard therapy, or no
treatment at all. But the benefit of receiving a new wonder drug
might be "psychological," either as a result of the hope generated by
getting the new drug or the attention lavished on the subject-patient
by the doctor; in addition, the chagrin at receiving no therapy or the
same old standard therapy might prove injurious to the ulcer patient.
Studies are therefore set up in such a way that the so-called control
group receives an inactive substitute made up to look and taste like
the active drug. Such a substitute is termed a *placebo*, though the British term *dummy* might be less confusing.

Clearly it would not be fair simply to select one patient to receive
the active drug and consign another to the inactive drug. Patients are
therefore chosen by lot (nowadays by computer) after being told they
will get either the active or the inactive drug. Because many observations have made clear that the extent of knowledge and enthusiasm
communicated to the patient by the investigator-physician heightens
the therapeutic effect of a drug (part of the placebo effect), controlled
trials are usually carried out double-blind. That is, neither the investigator-physician nor his patient-subjects know whether a given subject
is getting the active drug or the inactive placebo.

Placebo Healing in Controlled Trials

The results of double-blind controlled trials, of duodenal ulcer for
example, bring their own surprises; during a six-week period 50–60
percent of ulcers heal on placebo and about 70 percent on a specific
drug. An observer might conclude that the drug was effective and
could be approved by the Food and Drug Administration (FDA), but
he might have an interest in that 60 percent whose ulcer healed on
placebo. He might ask what such a result was telling physicians about
healing, medical arts, the need for medications, and so forth. He
might even wonder whether the healing effects of the drug could be
almost incidental to the symbolic nature of the meeting, however con-
strained by double-blind conventions, between the physician and the
patient.

It is curious that most physicians ignore the benefit of the placebo
in such trials, to focus on the difference between the placebo effect
and the active drug. In the first reported multicentric double-blind

study in the United States,[4] for example, patients who received placebo did almost as well as the patients who were given cimetidine. At the end of two weeks of treatment the ulcers had healed in 56 percent of patients receiving cimetidine and in only 37 percent of patients given placebo; at every other assessment period, up to six weeks, cimetidine and placebo were equally effective, judged by the proportion of patients in whom the ulcers had healed. While there have been a number of theories to explain these phenomena, little discussion has focused on the effect of the controlled trial itself. The authors of that study said, "If it is true that the high placebo healing incidence in our study is attributable to large antacid consumption, it might be expected that those placebo treated patients who took large amounts of antacid would exhibit a higher incidence of ulcer healing than did those patients who took less antacid."[5] In that paper, as in so many others, there was no consideration that the placebo might be specifically helpful, and little discussion of anything other than the medications given, a characteristic blind spot of most controlled clinical trials.

Can some of the benefit of placebo come simply from the careful, dedicated attention that patients in a study receive? The patient's hope that he is getting the active drug? I think so. At any rate the surprisingly high placebo response of patients in controlled trials for many disorders—angina pectoris, for example—makes it very hard to sort out the benefits of an active drug from those of a placebo.

Many sophisticated ramifications need not concern us now. For the present we need only agree that a placebo in a controlled clinical trial has a very different role from that in clinical practice. Because it is simply a substitute to keep the patient and the physician in ignorance of whether the patient-subject is receiving an active agent, the placebo is not given to assuage the patient or to cure his disease. In one sense then, this kind of placebo acts as a control for the time passing during the study and for the natural tendencies of the body to heal an ulcer crater. (In that sense the dummy is not inert: it simply lacks the putative pharmacological benefit of the drug under study.) To be sure, the reader may object, "But that is not what happens in real life!" True enough, in real life there is no study and we do not know how the observer, the very act of being observed, affects ulcer healing in the control subjects receiving the inactive agent. In clinical practice we do not know whether the physician has a healing effect. Just because we do not know how to frame a study of this question does not detract from its importance.

4. Binder, H. J., Cocco, A., Crossley, R. J., et al., Cimetidine in the treatment of duodenal ulcer, *Gastroenterology* 74:380–88, 1978.
5. Ibid.

Hawthorne Effect

The effect of an observer on any study has been called the Hawthorne effect.[6] It is very hard to control for the increased attention provided by a special study that brings its own benefit. Factory workers improve their efficiency as a direct result of the increased attention they are getting during an investigation, and the phenomenon is just as well known in medicine. A study using computers to help physicians with their diagnoses of acute abdominal emergencies showed increased skill of the physicians during the study.[7] The proportion of perforated appendices fell from 36 to 4 percent during the trial, but rose again to 20 percent after the study had ended. Even more interesting, simply telling doctors that their skills were being monitored led to improvement, but that data has apparently not been reported.

For now it is enough to distinguish the placebo given by the physician to help a patient from the placebo used in quite a different spirit in the controlled clinical trial. It may be pertinent to note, however, that very few commentators find any ethical or medical problem with the use of a placebo in clinical trials, unless an existing drug is believed to bring such great benefit that not to give it will harm the patient.[8]

Characteristics of a Clinical Trial

A controlled clinical trial has four usual features: (1) random assignment to therapeutic and control groups, (2) a double-blind structure, (3) placebo control (which maintains blindness and minimizes bias), and (4) a number of subjects large enough to satisfy statistical requirements specified beforehand.

Ethics of Placebo in Controlled Clinical Trials

When is it ethical to use a placebo in controlled clinical trials, and, when can such trials seem to benefit society more than the individual patient? There are no clear answers.[9] The physician-investigator wants good statistical data with sharp borders, and he knows that a

6. Roethlisberger, F. J. and Dickson, W. J., *Management and the workers*, Cambridge: Harvard University Press, 1939.

7. DeDombal, F. T., Leaper, D. J., Horrocks, J. C., et al., Human and computer-aided diagnosis of abdominal pain: Further report with emphasis on performance of clinicians, *Brit. Med. J.* 1:376–80, 1984.

8. Peterson, W. L., and Elashoff, J., Placebos in clinical trials of duodenal ulcer: The end of an era? *Gastroenterology* 79:585–88, 1980; Lam, S. K., A plea for the inclusion of a placebo group in duodenal ulcer trials, *Gastroenterology* 85:983, 1983.

9. Ritter, J. M., Placebo-controlled, double-blind clinical trials can impede medical progress, *Lancet* 1:1126–27, 1980; Pinto, H. A., Ethical guidelines for the use of placebos in clinical practice, thesis, Yale Univ. Sch. Med., 1983.

comparison with a placebo will give him the best chance to express the contrast between a new drug and the natural course of a disease. Yet no one thinks it right to use a placebo control for a disease in which current therapy is, say, effective in 25 percent of patients. Sachar and his colleagues suggest that a placebo is ethical only when the disease under study is one for which (1) no available therapy is effective or appropriate, (2) the placebo is also relatively effective, and (3) not treating has little adverse impact upon the patient.[10] In this last case we may ask what benefit any treatment brings.

But some observers have also asked whether placebo trials are ever ethical if patients are only going to have a fifty-fifty chance of receiving already effective therapy.[11] Clearly, in patients with Hodgkins disease, for example, where known therapy has proven so life-saving, a new therapeutic program must be compared to one already proven effective. But in the case of the routine, uncomplicated duodenal ulcer which is generally so benign, they ask whether placebo therapy in a trial could not be perfectly ethical. The answer is a mixed one. As the incidence of complications in patients receiving a placebo for duodenal ulcer is so small, even if it is twice as high as that of patients getting active therapy, a placebo controlled trial still seems ethical, at least in the United States. That is not the case in Britain, however, where physicians are so convinced of the dangers of the untreated duodenal ulcer that no current investigator will use placebo controlled trials. But even in the United States there are lingering doubts about whether a placebo trial is ethical if proven therapy has minimal side effects, such as is true of antacids or cimetidine, and the new drug has unknown side effects. Many prefer to compare a new drug with proven therapy, recognizing that such a comparison is much more difficult statistically than comparing a new drug with a placebo. A very large number of patients is required in the drug-drug comparison to show that a new drug brings only a very small improvement over current therapy; it is much easier statistically to compare a new drug with a placebo. To some extent this ethical dilemma is a social one: whether society should devote any share of its resources to proving the marginal superiority of the new drug over an old one or whether its energies and money could be better spent.[12]

The issue of informed consent in such clinical trials is much discussed and still unresolved. Much attention has been focused on the differences between a patient and a subject, and on the tensions a

10. Sachar, D., Placebo-controlled clinical trials in gastroenterology, *Amer. J. Gastroenterol.* 79:913–17, 1984.
11. Peterson and Elashoff, Placebos in clinical trials.
12. Dollery, C. T., A bleak outlook for placebos (and for science), *Eur. J. Clin. Pharmacol.* 15:219–21, 1979.

physician sometimes feels when carrying out clinical studies on his own patients, uncertain whether he is advancing his own interests or theirs. Entire books have been devoted to the topic, but here I shall simply ask whether it is ever possible to get from a patient with an acute illness valid informed consent to any kind of randomized therapeutic trial. Can the forty-year-old man in the coronary care unit (CCU) choose not to participate in a study designed to assess limiting the size of a myocardial infarct when his doctor leans over the bedrail to ask him? But such considerations will not detain us here.

It is probably easier to specify when placebo controlled trials are *not* indicated: (1) when death or disability is a possibility if no treatment is given, (2) when alternative therapy is effective, or (3) when the experimental drug or procedure is already known to be effective if the study is designed simply to assess the exact magnitude of benefit.

Let us turn momentarily from peptic ulcer, which has provided so many useful lessons, to the natural history of Crohn's disease. Meyers and Janowitz have surveyed recent controlled trials in this disorder to conclude that placebo trials give useful information about the natural history of disease, tempering physicians' enthusiasm for active therapy.[13] They emphasize that "a patient sick enough to require treatment on an ambulatory basis can get better with no specific drug therapy."

Although making such a statement may betray bald confidence in what physicians think they can do, and—in the therapeutic triumphalism of the 1980s—an obliviousness to the healing power of nature, their assessment provides an important reminder. In four months 25–40 percent of patients with Crohn's disease receiving only placebo therapy in a controlled trial improved enough so that they could be considered to have gone into remission. Even more salutary a reminder is their finding that three-quarters of all patients who went into remission in a controlled clinical trial stayed well without specific maintenance therapy for over a year. Indeed almost two-thirds of patients (63 percent) continued well at the end of two years. They remind us what physicians used to know, that even patients with Crohn's disease get better without active intervention. Their conclusion should "temper our enthusiasm for the medicines we are currently using with their limited efficacy and their known toxicity."[14] Of course all patients in these studies had continuing guaranteed physician contact, support, and enthusiasm, and, as always, this may have

13. Meyers, S., and Janowitz, H. D., The "natural history" of Crohn's disease: An analytic review of the placebo lesson, *Gastroenterology* 87:1189–92, 1984.
14. Ibid.

had much to do with the patients getting and staying well. But, of course, it may not.

At any event the studies suggest what many experienced clinicians have held for a long time, that continuing contact with patients with Crohn's disease is therapeutic. The physician may not feel that he is doing very much for his patients, but somehow the active keeping in touch seems to keep things under control. Patients must realize this too, even if unconsciously, for a number of people have told me that they want another appointment "anyway" in three or four months. I assume that kind of medical contact provides a placebic therapy even if it is not intended in that way.

Importance of Placebo Controls

In duodenal ulcer trials the absence of a placebo control may lead to accepting as effective drugs which in truth may not be very much more active than a placebo. The healing rate on placebo for duodenal ulcer craters in controlled clinical trials runs from 20 percent in London to 70 percent in Switzerland.[15] In the United States it ranges from 50 to 60 percent. A very interesting study was conducted in the United Kingdom a few years ago.[16] An anti-ulcer drug was compared to a placebo in a trial carried out in Dundee and in London. The study was identical at both hospitals, but the healing rates for placebo were quite different: in Dundee 73 percent of ulcers healed on a placebo, in contrast to only 44 percent in London. The reasons for the differences in the healing rates in the two centers were unclear to the observers, who wondered whether there was a difference in the patients, in the doctors taking care of the patients, or in someone's expectation of cure. A study in the United States foreshadowed this observation.[17] In one hospital Littman found that antacids relieved pain 79 percent of the time, but in another hospital the same antacids were effective only 17 percent of the time. In one hospital placebos gave relief to 45 percent of the patients, but in another only 25 percent were helped. In both the British and American studies the experimental design, definition of terms, and criteria were the same, but the re-

15. Gudjonsson, B., and Spiro, H. M., Response to placebos in ulcer disease, *Amer. J. Med.* 65:399–402, 1978; Blum, A. L., Is placebo the ideal anti-ulcer drug? in *Peptic ulcer disease*, Bianchi, G., and Bardhan, K. D., eds., New York: Raven Press, 1982, pp. 57–61); Fordtran, J. S., Placebos, antacids, and cimetidine for duodenal ulcer, *NEJM* 298:1081–83, 1978.

16. MacDonald, A. J., Peden, N. R., Hayton, R., et al., Symptom relief and the placebo effect in the trial of an antipeptic drug, *Gut* 21:323–26, 1980.

17. Littman, A., Welch, R., Fruin, R. C., et al., Controlled trials of aluminum hydroxide gels for peptic ulcer, *Gastroenterology* 73:6–10, 1977.

sponses were different, suggesting there are fundamental differences in responses to placebo as well as to therapy. In France Sarles also found that different physicians had different placebo healing rates and that these rates tended to be fairly constant over time.[18]

The British observers decided that the differences had something to do with an expectation of complete cure, and I suppose by implication felt that the physicians must have been responsible for that. The reasons are not as important as the problems that may arise if a drug is compared only to another drug already known to be active. For whatever reason the population studied may consist of more rapid responders than is generally the case, and so a drug may be equal to cimetidine, which is the current standard, and yet not really be very much better than a placebo.[19] Moreover, there are major statistical problems in comparing a new drug against the standard of cimetidine: Lam suggests that a sample size of at least seven hundred is necessary to avoid false conclusions about the efficacy of any new drug.[20] Clearly, now that peptic ulcer is so readily treated by the H2 blockers, enlisting seven hundred patients for control trials is not easy. These are important questions. Already several careful observers, both statisticians and clinicians, have suggested that it is easier not to bother with placebo trials.[21] Attempts to reduce the number of patients receiving placebo in controlled trials are underway.

PLACEBO AS THERAPY

There have been many changes in the use of, and lengthy discussions about the term *placebo*. In 1946 a very important conference on the use of placebos in treatment was published, but so obscurely as rarely to be referenced.[22] Although a definition of placebo was not specifically given, the implication of the physicians in this conference, which deserves rereading because it foreshadows most future discussions, was that the placebo pill was pharmacologically inactive. Harry Gold defined it as "a chemical device for psychotherapy, . . . largely devoid of pharmacological properties."

18. Sarles, H., Camatte, R., and Sahel, J., A study of the variations in the response regarding duodenal ulcers when treated with placebo by different investigators, *Digestion* 16:289–92, 1977.

19. Spiro, H. M., H2 Blockers: How safe and how effective? *J. Clin. Gastroenterology* 5(suppl. 1):143–47, 1983.

20. Lam, A plea.

21. Peterson and Elashoff, Placebos in clinical trials.

22. Wolff, H. G., DuBois, F., Gold, H., Cornell Conferences on Therapy: Uses of placebo in therapy, *New York J. Med.* 46:1718–27, 1946.

Most commentators follow Shapiro, who broadly defined it as any therapy *deliberately or unknowingly* used for its nonspecific, psychologic, or psychoprophylactic effect.[23]

Later Shapiro developed a more extensive definition of placebo in his 1971 review: "A placebo is defined as any therapy (or that component of any therapy) that is deliberately used for its non-specific psychologic or psychophysiologic effect, or that is used for its presumed specific effect on a patient, symptom, or illness, but which, unknown to *patient and therapist*, is without specific activity for the condition being treated" (emphasis added).

Sissela Bok's definition of a placebo as a drug "which has no specific effect . . . on a patient's condition, but which can have powerful psychological effects"[24] seems to me to fall wide of the mark in that Bok explicitly separates "psychological" effects from "physical" ones. Bond defines as a placebo "any therapeutic procedure . . . which is objectively without specific activity for the condition treated."[25] The problem comes in how to define "objective." H. Brody, a philosopher as well as clinician, who has provided a philosophical and ethical framework for placebo therapy, defines a placebo as "a form of medical therapy, or an intervention designed to simulate medical therapy, that is believed to be without specific activity for the condition being treated and that is used . . . for its symbolic effect."[26]

Grunbaum, a philosopher and logician, has dealt at length with the logical problems in defining a placebo and especially with the terms *specific* and *nonspecific* as applied to the effect of a placebo.[27] He calls it misleading to treat an effect of therapy as nonspecific simply because we do not know how it works. The effect of a placebo can be precisely defined, what is at issue is how it works, what factors are responsible. Grunbaum would substitute "unspecified" for "nonspecific," and most physicians less rigorous would understand "unknown" factors. The effect of a placebo, as I shall emphasize, is characteristic: it relieves pain. We will examine the mechanisms responsible for that pain relief and where the mechanism is to be looked for below. With that caveat, I like Brody's definition and will follow it, emphasizing the importance of intent. When we come to evaluate

23. Shapiro, A. K., Factors contributing to the placebo effect, *Amer. J. Psychiatry* 18:73–88, 1964.

24. Bok, S., *Lying: Moral choice in public and private life*, New York: Pantheon Books, 1978, p. 61.

25. Bond, M., *Pain: Its nature, analysis and treatment*, New York: Churchill Livingstone, 1979, p. 135.

26. Brody, H., The lie that heals: The ethics of giving placebos, *Ann. Intern. Med.* 97:112–18, 1982.

27. Grunbaum, A., The placebo concept, *Behav. Res. Therapy* 19:157–67, 1981.

the effect of placebos on disease, the physician's intent will prove important.

Let me define science and intuition as I will use the terms throughout this book. *Science*, the process whereby new knowledge is created, gives us "objective knowledge of nature," which is quantitative and verifiable. The scientific method depends upon observation and experimentation, and requires agreement about the observations; therefore science relies on sensory organs, largely the eyes, and upon physical instruments. Beyond experimentation, manipulation, and control, the scientific method requires verification by others. The *OED* defines science as "a branch of study which is concerned either with a connected body of demonstrated truths or with observed facts . . . and which includes trustworthy methods for the discovery of new truths within its own domain. . . . Those branches of study that relate to the phenomena of the material universe and their laws." Bertrand Russell offers a definition of science in *Religion and Science*: "Science is the attempt to discover by means of observation, and reasoning based upon it, first, particular facts about the world and then laws connecting facts with one another and (in fortunate cases) making it possible to predict future occurrences."[28] Later he adds, "Science does not include art, or friendship, or various other valuable elements in life. . . . Science can tell us much about the *means* of realizing our desires, but it cannot say that one desire is preferable to another."[29] Montague distinguished intuition from science in the following way:

> We might take as an example of the elemental interest romantic love and judgement of faith on which it is based. It would surely be a vain and preposterous undertaking to discover one's true sweetheart by accepting the authority of others, by using deductive reasoning and calculation, by cold-blooded empirical analysis of her perceivable qualities, or by considering the extent to which she might be a practical utility. . . . True friendship is certainly not based upon either calculation or utility, but upon the direct appeal to our sympathies and affections.[30]

Intuition, on the other hand, is what we know by immediate apprehension, at a glance, without conscious activity. For my purposes it is knowledge which is nonmeasurable, nonquantifiable. The *OED* defines intuition as "immediate knowledge. . . . The immediate apprehension of an object by the mind without the intervention of any rea-

28. Russell, B., *Religion and science*, London: Oxford University Press, 1935, p. 8.
29. Ibid., p. 175.
30. Montague, W. P., quoted by Titus, H. H. and Smith, M. S., *Living issues in philosophy*, 6th ed., New York: Van Nostrand, 1974, p. 242.

distinguish between belief and intent when look-
giving a placebo. Does the physician give a pla-
t he is giving an active agent when he is not, or
e an inactive drug?

the physician and what is in his mind when he
he relief of pain physicians usually try the weak-
first. They will prescribe aspirin before codeine,
rol, and so forth, even for the patient who is dy-
rge extent physicians think of placebos as weak
with few side effects. If they give them at all,
placebos for pain or anxiety rather than taking
m. From this perspective, the physician may give
allenge, or ransom.

) AS GIFT

generous mode the physician gives a pill to re-
a complaint, particularly if he believes the pa-
without merit, that is, if he suspects that the
bjective explanation. He does not want to give
drug, for a pain which has no detectable origin,
mpted to use a placebo to relieve anxiety. He
nhances the awareness of pain or other symp-
ield to the symbolic assuaging of a pill. This aim
s, even if it is paternalistic, and falls into the cat-

) AS CHALLENGE

r, a physician will use a placebo as a challenge,
tlet to the patient, to prove to himself and even
patient is wrong. When the placebo is given in
tionship, it is being abused, symbols are wrongly
elieve, poor medical judgment is exercised.
ost likely recipients of a placebo as challenge
ter an operation who continues to ask for pain
staff thinks he should, (2) the patient who has
upon narcotics to relieve pain or discomfort of
deemed addicted, or (3) the patient who com-
nhappy, and who is always asking for some-
tice, too, physicians often use placebos as a

win, J. M., and Vogel, A. V., Knowledge and use of place-
rses, *Ann. Intern. Med.* 91:106–10, 1979.

soning process." *Webster's* which does not offer a useful definition of
science, at least in my new *International Dictionary* (1925), defines intuition as "direct of immediate knowing, whether mystical, percep-
tional, intellectual or moral, contrasted with speculative, reflective or
mediate knowing." For thinking about the placebo I like Bergson's
depiction of intuition and intelligence as pointing in opposite directions. For Bergson intelligence is the tool that science uses to deal
with matter, with things and quantitative relationships, whereas intuition is inward, immediate, and a vision of reality: "The former toward inert matter, the latter toward life."[31]

Using "mysticism" as his term for intuition, Russell suggests the following contrast:

> When a man of science tells us the result of an experiment, he also
> tells us how the experiment was performed; others can repeat it,
> and if the result is not confirmed it is not accepted as true. . . . The
> mystic himself may be certain that he *knows*, and has no need of sci-
> entific tests but those who are asked to accept his testimony will
> subject it to the same kind of scientific tests as those applied to men
> who say they have been to the North Pole. . . . The chief argument
> in favour of the mystics is their agreement with each other. . . . I
> cannot admit any method of arriving at truth except that of sci-
> ence, but in the realm of the emotions I do not deny the value of
> the experiences which have given rise to religion.[32]

In *Mysticism and Logic* Russell had already attacked mysticism, "the belief in insight as against discursive analytic knowledge: the belief in a
way of wisdom, sudden, penetrating coercive, which is contrasted
with the slow and fallible study of outward appearance by science
relying wholly upon the senses."[33]

Arguing from the other side, Buber gives a rich interpretation of
intuition: If we want to do today's work and prepare tomorrow's with
clear sight, then we must develop in ourselves and in the next generation a gift which lives in man's inwardness as a Cinderella, one day to
be a princess. Some call it intuition, but that is not a wholly unambigu-
ous concept. I prefer the name "imagining the real," for in its essential being this gift is not a looking at the other, but a bold swinging,
demanding the most intensive stirring of one's being, into the life of
the other.[34]

For the scientist intuition can simply turn out to be "serendip-

31. Bergson, H., *Creative Evolution*, New York: Modern Library, 1944, p. 194.
32. Russell, *Religion and science*, p. 178.
33. Russell, B., *Mysticism and logic*, Garden City: Doubleday, 1957.
34. Buber, M., The William Alanson White Memorial Lectures, 4th series: Distance and relation, *Psychiatry* 20:97–113, 1957.

ity,"[35] the readiness of the prepared mind to grasp a new opportunity. For the neurobiologist that will mean circuits all wired up and ready to go, given the proper calcium influx or program. But for one retired chemist and physician musing over the discoveries that had come to him early in his career, intuition was the "welcome stranger . . . , essentially wild . . . , invisible, inaudible, and imponderable. It is not subject to scientific testing because it is not amenable to scientific procedures; certainly it cannot be summoned at will."[36]

There is so much talk in medicine about truth and facts that it is worthwhile looking at the *OED* definition of *fact*, "something that has really occurred or is actually the case . . . a particular truth known by actual observation or authentic testimony, as opposed to what is merely inferred . . . a datum of experience as distinguished from the conclusions that may be based upon it." *Truth* is defined almost as a synonym: "conformity with fact, agreement with reality . . . The fact or facts; the actual state of the case, the matter or circumstances as it really is."

Let me emphasize that it is not my purpose even to attempt to enter into the distinctions between science and intuition which such profound thinkers have considered. I simply want to lay out the distinctions or dichotomy that I am setting out when I talk about science as knowledge which is quantifiable and intuition which is not. It is, I suggest, the contrast of the two elements in humans, intelligence and emotion, or on a more practical level, physics and poetry. I am suggesting that the poetic imagination is as important to medical practice as science. Yet in looking at the claims of intuition of alternative medicine, for example, we must be scientific. If two claims are made for cure of a disease, one by a faith healer and the other by an investigator, we must judge both claims on a scientific basis. In that regard Russell suggested: "What I do wish to maintain—and it is here that the scientific attitude becomes imperative—is that insight, untested and unsupported, is an insufficient guarantee of truth, in spite of the fact that much of the most important truth is first suggested by its means."[37]

When we look at alternative medicine, when we examine the placebo and its effects, we must remember the basis of scientific validation: "Instinct, intuition, or insight is what first leads to the beliefs which subsequent reason confirms or confutes."[38]

35. Cannon, W. B., Gains from serendipity, In *The way of an investigator*, New York: Norton, 1945.

36. Jacobs, H. R., Intuition: The welcome stranger, *Perspectives in Biology and Medicine* 24:457–66, 1981.

37. Russell, *Mysticism and logic*, p. 11.

38. Ibid., p. 12.

It is important to
ing at the physician
cebo in the belief th
does he intend to gi

Let us look first a
gives a placebo. For
est therapeutic agen
codeine before dem
ing of cancer. To a
pain-relieving agen
physicians prescribe
any more dramatic a
a placebo as a gift, c

PLACEB

In the best or mo
lieve pain or to trea
tient's complaints a
complaints have no
demerol, an addictin
and so he may be t
knows that anxiety
toms and that it may
can be called genero
egory of gift.

PLACEB

Sometimes, howe
to throw down a gau
to the patient that th
such an adversary re
manipulated, and, I
In a hospital the
are: (1) the patient a
relief longer than th
become so dependen
any origin that he is
plains, who remains
thing.[3] In office pra

ways sub
themselv
such pow
or near tl
to other
partly fro
the awesc
could do
reputatio
ous disea
not forth
themselv
they aro
doctor c
wish tha
cared. G
ity of te
Shapiro
saying th
therape

1. Ar
Mechanic,
2. Sh
Dis., 130:
practice:
94, 1982.

3. Goodwin, J. S., Goo
bos by house officers and n

challenge to prove that the pain can be relieved by a placebo and therefore that it has no important origin: "See, if a sugar pill has helped you, it is all in your mind!"

Sometimes the physician gives an active drug for what he takes to be a nonspecific symptom in the hope that the complaint will go away, and that, having treated it with an active drug, he can then ascribe the symptom to a real disease or at the least to a physiological mechanism which has gone awry. Cimetidine is one of the commonest drugs currently used in this manner.[4] It reduces acid secretion by blocking receptors on the parietal cell responsible for acid secretion; it speeds up the healing of peptic ulcer and relieves its pain. (Placebos also relieve the pain of peptic ulcer, but that need not concern us now.) But many physicians who are averse to deceiving their patients reason that giving cimetidine to the patient with "existential" pain, coming from his life circumstances, may make it go away, so that they and their patients can be satisfied and a confrontation with any emotional issues avoided. Obviously, giving an active drug to a patient with a poorly definable pain may give placebic relief, that is, it may work through its symbolic rather than its pharmacological value; but the pain relief from such an active drug makes the physician feel less guilty than giving a placebo. Used in this way, cimetidine falls into the category of an impure placebo.

PLACEBO AS RANSOM

Finally, to get rid of demanding patients, as a sop or pacifier, and too often with real hostility, physicians may use a placebo as pure deception. One study emphasized how house officers in hospital practice gave placebos to the hostile, demanding patient who has become too difficult to deal with or complains too much.[5] Giving a placebo to such a patient brands him as a "crock" and spares everyone dealing with him from any need to try to help or to understand. A placebo so given often symbolizes the agreement of the staff that the patient is beyond their help and concern:

We found that placebos were rarely prescribed—about one prescription per year per physician—but that, in almost every instance in which a placebo was prescribed, the physician and staff were having great difficulty relating to a particular patient. Physicians and nurses may need to prove that such difficult and unlikeable patients are not really ill because they need to believe that they

4. Schade, R. R., and Donaldson, R. M., How physicians use cimetidine, *NEJM* 304:1281–84, 1981.

5. Goodwin, Goodwin, and Vogel, Knowledge and use of placebos.

would never become so angry and frustrated with a genuinely ill person.[6]

When we examine ethical justifications for placebo we will see that giving a placebo as ransom is deemed justifiable if it is intended to be the first step in a therapeutic alliance or in moving the patient toward improvement.

BELIEF

The foregoing analysis leads me to suggest that the intent of the physician will prove an important factor in the ethical appropriateness of a placebo. Placebos benefit patients, however, regardless of the mood in which the doctor prescribes them, and that is one of its wonders.

To some extent, of course, we will have to judge the intent of a physician by what he knows. The more knowledgeable the physician, the more likely he is to recognize that sometimes a medicine is really only acting as a placebo. The less well-trained physician, out of ignorance or innocence, may believe that his pills work by a specific pharmacological mechanism.

Even today the benefit of many active drugs depends in part upon the shared faith of physician and patient, but to be a placebo by my definition a drug must be given by a physician who believes that the drug he prescribes is inactive. Grunbaum uses the term "intentional" for such an action, and contrasts it with "inadvertent" placebo, giving a worthless inactive drug in the belief that it is effective.[7] That puts him and me in the difficult position of saying that the same drug which is a placebo for one physician may not be for another. In other words, a sophisticated physician may know that a drug is useless and give it only as a placebo, but a less informed physician gives the same drug convinced of its efficacy. To be sure, suggestion is present in both prescriptions, but the first physician is using a placebo, the second is not. While the drug itself may be inactive and bring benefit only by virtue of the physician-patient relationship, both erroneously believing in it, such a transaction does not fall under the narrow definition offered here. The ignorant physician unwittingly brings about a placebo response, but in this discussion I will concentrate on the physician who knows that he is giving an inactive drug. The good physician knows the power of his role.

A study by the National Institutes of Health has reaffirmed the

6. Ibid.
7. Grunbaum, A., The placebo concept, *Behav. Res. Therapy* 19:157–67, 1981.

contribution of the faith of the placebo-giver in enhancing the effectiveness of placebo pain relief.[8] When clinicians expected their patients to improve more on one placebo than on others, those patients reported significantly more pain relief.

An unnamed editorial writer for the *Lancet* asked in this regard: "Here is a puzzle for medical ethicists: why is it deceitful to give a placebo if a large element of modern therapeutics is no better than placebo? Is the gullibility of a good-hearted doctor preferable to (and more ethical than) the skepticism of one whose prescription is pharmacologically inert, when the results are the same?"[9]

EARLY USE OF "PLACEBO" BY PHYSICIANS

Physicians of the past, it is said, gave placebos in the belief that they were giving active medicines. It is often asserted that early and primitive medicine is only the history of the placebo. However true that may be, it should not be taken as an indictment, for the role of the physician has loomed large in history. After all, Plato and Aristotle turned to the physician and the medical method as one model for philosophy.[10] They must have seen some value in the profession and not found it consistently humbug. It is hard to conjecture why so many observers deride medical history until modern times as only the history of the placebo. Such critics apparently accept only the biomedical-mechanical model of disease, and consider the caring role much less important than the curing role.

Before the development of rational scientific therapy, much of what physicians achieved, of course, must have depended on the physician-patient relationship, along with their time-tested empiric remedies. Although many patients died of their diseases, some lived, but it surely cannot have been only the statistical quirks for which physicians took credit. They could only rarely cure diseases; but they comforted, relieved, and helped by being caretakers. What they did must have satisfied many, unless only diseases of biological origin are held as important. Moreover, if the intent of the physician figures into the definition of the placebo, then surely some physicians gave harmless (or harmful) pills or potions unwittingly in the faith they worked. If we define the placebo, as I do, in part by the *intent* of the

8. Gracely, R. H., Dubner, R., Deeter, W. R., et al., Clinicians' expectations influence placebo analgesia, *Lancet* 1:43, 1985.

9. Anon., Shall I please? *Lancet* 2:1465–66, 1983.

10. Lloyd, G. E., The role of medical and biological analogies in Aristotle's ethics, *Phronesis* 13:68–83, 1968.

physician, such wide-ranging disparagement of medical practices of the past are not easy to accept.

THE PHYSICIAN: HEALER OR CONDUIT?

Today, of course, most medicines are given with apparent scientific rationale. Physicians rely much less on themselves as therapeutic agents, but instead have faith in the medicines available to them.

What about the physician as healer? That idea has come in for much criticism over the past few decades. Physicians are embarrassed to consider themselves as healers and relegate any such notion to a fictitious charisma. The more medical science advances, the more the art of medicine seems to decline. The reason for this, of course, is that physicians see themselves as those who cure disease, not as healers of persons. For that reason physicians contrast what they can do for the patient with pneumonia without antibiotics to the cure by penicillin, with an obvious answer.

A recurrent theme of this book, but a paradoxical one, is that the more medical science does for disease, the less physicians seem to do for patients. As hospitals have become corporate enterprises with battalions of staff wielding arms against disease, the individual physician counts for less in the hospital. Still, even in the out-patient department or in his office, where a physician could count for so much more, he relies ever increasingly on the diagnostic and therapeutic technology which he learned in medical school and in residency rather than on the comfort his personal skill can assure.

It might seem that reliance on therapeutic technology characterizes only university hospitals, but as thousands of well-trained, technologically able physicians have moved out to community hospitals, those hospitals look very little different from their university counterparts in the application of technology to medical problems. Indeed physicians at community hospitals prove even more enthusiastically adept than their university counterparts. "When someone is dying," a friend in such a hospital remarked, "they call for the priest to give last rites and the cardiologist to pass a Swan (Ganz catheter) at the same time."

Physicians in Hospital

In the hospital technological advances have improved the outcome of most acute medical diseases, but specialization has proceeded so far that most practicing physicians have little to do with such technology. Respirators, catheters, pacemakers, and much other paraphernalia are essential life-savers, but they require the special attention of an acolyte-technician or physician-specialist. Intensive care units (ICUs),

CCUs, and a whole panoply of special interests have divided and sub-divided the hospital into specialized duchies or turfs, each with its own master.

Just look at the implication of those metaphors. Duchy suggests a duke with absolute power, and turf a dog defending with his bark and his teeth his living space or, in its later revival, a youthful gang member defending his space with knife or gun. But those are the words I have heard administrators and other chiefs use in relation to current "battles."

Most big hospitals have little room for the general physician without specific technical skill, who simply takes care of patients. Increasingly even the specialist turns his patients over to a team. Far from criticizing this division I applaud it as the only way to give the critically ill the benefits of modern technology. But these arrangements may be affecting the physician's view of himself. Even the cardiologist, the very prototype of the technologically skilled specialist, is often at a loss to deal with ever-changing new apparatus a few years after his training, a poignant example of how developing technology so quickly makes physicians' skills obsolete. Before the development of cardiac intensive care technology, for example, an earnest physician might sit some hours by the bed of his patient with a heart attack watching for arrhythmias or other doleful turn. Now, as soon as the patient with chest pain comes to the emergency room, he is turned over to the monitors in the CCU, to the television screens, CCU nurses, resident physicians, and CCU specialists. This is all to the good, (assuming, for the moment, that CCUs save lives), for these personnel are far more skilled in wielding the new and constantly changing tools than the practicing office-based cardiologist. If this is true of the general cardiologist, it is even more true of the general physician, who has become simply a guide to the technology which gives better care than ever to patients with acute disease. It is then no coincidence that the growth of science and technology in medicine has led to skepticism about what an individual physician can do. Yet it is paradoxical that the more powerless the individual physician becomes, the louder the clamor for family physicians, for guides, for friends.

Of course even hospital-based physicians can be much more than simple conduits of power. Studies from the 1960s suggest how much old-fashioned encouragement can do and how powerful an agent the physician-as-person can be. Anesthetists at the Massachusetts General Hospital studied two groups of patients who were about to undergo elective intraabdominal operations.[11] One group was not given any

11. Egbert, L. D., Battit, G. E., Welch, C. E. et al., Reduction in post-operative pain by encouragement and instruction of patients, *NEJM* 270:825–27, 1964.

specific instructions or information about postoperative pain, while the other was told what to expect and how to allay such pain: "The presentation was given in a manner of enthusiasm and confidence; the patients were not informed that we were conducting a study. The surgeons, not knowing which patients were receiving special care, continued their practices as usual." Anesthetists visited the special patients after the operation to encourage them with results that might have been expected: the amount of narcotics required postoperatively was reduced by half: "The anesthetist who understands his patient and who believes that each patient is 'his' patient ceases to be merely a clever technician in the operating room." Whether the effect is placebo or communication, whether a physician or some other person could achieve the same reduction in the amount of narcotics required, is unimportant. Such simple observations underline what physicians used to know and have forgotten, that they can do something for their patients, that the good physician can do something to help all of his patients, if only he will try.

Physicians in Office

In the late-twentieth-century hospital patients are likely to have serious diseases of biological origin that are easily detected. In this battlefield against death physicians receive their medical training for future practice. In the office, on the other hand, or in the out-patient clinics, diseases are more chronic and complaints less likely to have a biologically detectable origin, at least at present. From ancient times physicians have been aware of the importance of the psychological distress which accounts for so many visits to the doctor. In modern times estimates of the frequency of emotional factors in out-patients vary enormously depending upon what the observer defines as functional disease. For Cabot at the Massachusetts General Hospital in 1904, 47 percent of patients who attended the medical clinic had functional disease, by which he meant constipation, dyspepsia, debility, apprehension, and the like.[12] Sixty years later studies in the same hospital suggested that in 84 percent of patients psychological distress was the major impetus in their coming to the medical clinic.[13] The later study also indicated the importance of psychological distress in precipitating the decision to get help, something any practitioner awakened in the middle of the night could have attested to without a study.

Many complaints in office practice turn out to have no biologically

12. Cabot, R. C., Suggestions for re-organization of hospital outpatient departments, *Maryland Med. J.* 50:81, 1907.
13. Stoeckle, J. D., Zola, I. K., and Davidson, G. E., The quantity and significance of psychological distress in medical patients, *J. Chr. Dis.* 17:959–70, 1964.

detectable origin. The problem is that in the attempt to avoid what is widely known as a "Type 1 error"—dismissing the patient who is actually ill[14]—most physicians begin with the assumption that most complaints have an organic biological origin. This avoids personal or professional embarrassment as well as expensive malpractice lawsuits. What are known as "Type 2 errors"—accepting the notion that a patient has a disease when in fact he does not—are usually judged by most physicians as less harmful. Relying on symptom relief somewhat more than is now popular might reduce the Type 2 errors.

Even in their offices many physicians have come to see themselves as simple conduits of more powerful forces, of technology and pills, and have come to regard themselves as passive agents except in helping their patients to make choices. In part that is the result of medical school and hospital training, but in part it is one consequence of the patient autonomy movement. The aging physician inevitably falling behind in developing technology used to base himself ever more securely and supremely in his office, where he treated aging people developing chronic disorders, and turned patients with acute problems over to colleagues more recently trained and more comfortable in the hospital. Behind his desk, in his office he reigned in retreat, giving advice and helping patients to decide about their lives. Now, however, the physician has come under attack as paternalistic. What the physician before took as his duty is now seen as reprehensibly authoritarian. The practicing physician does not always understand modern technology—and does not need to—but his penchant for advice-giving has also come under criticism. It sometimes seems that the physician has little left to feel good about.

Effect of Controlled Clinical Trials

Controlled clinical trials have contributed to the growth of the conviction that the physician has no therapeutic effect as a person, but is simply a conduit of pills or procedures. As we have already seen, in the controlled clinical trial the placebo provides a control for the passage of time, simply to show that time—and observation—effects some cures. Holding all physicians as equal in a trial implicitly suggests, however, that the physician himself does not matter. That is not the intent of the trials, which are the best way so far devised to assess the value of a drug or treatment, but I fear that one of their unintended side effects is the conviction that physicians as therapists are all the same.

We may know that manual dexterity varies, that one surgeon will be more skilled than another; we may suspect that the ability to inter-

14. Feinstein, A. R., *Clinical Epidemiology*, Philadelphia: Saunders, 1985.

pret X-rays and other images depends on more than training, but psychiatrists more than most recognize that the ability to heal may vary from one physician to another. Yet at least one controlled trial of ulcer therapy has suggested that physicians vary in their placebo or healing capacities and that they are characterized by differences that are no less real for being hard to evaluate.[15]

There must be as much variation in the physician who attends as in the patient who responds. In ulcer healing trials, for example, I find it difficult to concede that it is only the characteristics of the crater and the disease which influence healing. A British study showing a markedly better response to placebo in Dundee than in London suggests otherwise.[16] The study by Sarles in Marseilles showing that different doctors engendered different healing rates of duodenal ulcer was also important in the preliminary finding that the placebo-healing rates for doctors remained unchanged over time.[17] I would have preferred to believe that with age and equanimity the charismatic healing of physicians would have grown. At any rate I suspect that the personality and qualities of the patient-subject and of the physician are equally important. Because we can measure the dimensions of the ulcer, we should not ignore the patient who has the ulcer or the doctor who treats it. Does an angry doctor, or a hostile or cold one, slow the healing process? Change the placebo effect? In all our considerations of the placebo, we must not forget that there are vast differences in the physicians who give them as well as in their conscious motives.

Charismatic Healing

Such a prize is placed upon objective measurable data that any benefit from laying on of hands has become embarrassing to physicians and demeaning to patients. Using a placebo makes many physicians feel guilty—or ashamed—at their nonscientific attitude. Burt comments:

> The rigor with which the placebo effect must be eliminated before any medical intervention can be viewed as efficacious points to two critical aspects of contemporary physicians' views of themselves: first, that the magical "laying on of hands" which had such prominence in earlier physicians' views of their calling is now widely seen as inconsistent with the highest aspiration of medical practice. . . .

15. MacDonald, A. J., Peden, N. R., Hayton, R., et al., Symptom relief and the placebo effect in the trial of an antipeptic drug, *Gut* 21:323–26, 1980.

16. Ibid.

17. Sarles, H., Camatte, R., and Sahel, J., A study of the variation in the response regarding duodenal ulcer when treated with placebo by different investigators, *Digestion* 16:289–92, 1977.

Normative valuation of objectivity in the modern practice of medicine have not only affected physicians' views of themselves. These facts have also dramatically altered physicians' views of their interpersonal relations with patients. . . . A physician who aspires to scientific objectivity can properly assert that, insofar as the efficacy of his therapy depends on his personal will, he has transgressed the norms of his profession.[18]

As Burt has pointed out, the healing power of charismatic medicine demands a double-blind trial, but that will be hard to arrange given current views of informed consent.

A definition of *charisma* is useful at this point, as the word has achieved a considerable popularity in medical circles. The *OED* defines *charisma* as "a free gift or favour specially vouchsafed by God; a grace, a talent." In secular medical circles charismatic healing probably refers to the personal authority of the physician and any benefit that brings.

The Physician's Self-Image

Still, how much physicians vary in their charismatic healing, and why, needs consideration. How much the physician's image of himself plays a role in his therapeutic effectiveness deserves more thought. What model or metaphor he has chosen may be crucial. The metaphor of physician as father (or mother), as scientist, or as soldier all have different implications and must engage different relationships between physician and patient, and between one physician and his different patients. If the physician sees himself as powerless and the placebo as useless, he may give one in the spirit of a challenge, no matter how comforting his demeanor or frame of mind. The metaphor may not even be experienced, but may remain an unconscious controlling force in his practice. Lipkin has emphasized that the physician cannot avoid the placebo effect, but he can make it helpful or destructive depending on his own attitudes.[19]

The physician who sees himself as a scientist searching out the facts, betting on the one in one hundred shot will find his duty to the patient to be as thorough and as objective as possible. The physician whose metaphor for his relationship to his patients is father will have a far different view of his duty. Clinical research has been compared by some participants to the Olympics. That view of medicine as a sport implies a certain competitiveness, as anyone who has watched the last two minutes of college football games will appreciate. The

18. Burt, R. A., *Taking care of strangers*, New York: Free Press, 1979, pp. 106, 116.
19. Lipkin, M., Suggestion and healing, *Persp. Biol. Med.* 28:121–26, 1984.

burst of energy with which the two teams attempt to win in the final seconds suggests that the metaphor of the Olympics might carry over into the diagnostic process, to effect on the body of the patient the one in one hundred victory. In that regard, will the physician who has been a football player in his formative years bring different skills or even ethical viewpoints to the medical enterprise than one who has been a chess player? A long-distance runner? A poet?

The Physician as Active Agent

The idea that the physician brings very little benefit to his patient and his patient's disease except as he brings him pills and procedures has been growing since modern medicine began to become scientific and focus on disease rather than on the patient. In an address to the American College of Physicians in 1937, "The Doctor Himself as a Therapeutic Agent," Houston laid out the growing confidence of physicians that "with the name of Pasteur we associate an increasing rapid acceleration in our emancipation from the sway of the placebo."[20] For modern physicians Pasteur plays the same role as Galileo for the physicist. Houston had scanned the pages of Hippocrates "in vain for any treatments of specific value." All the medicines used up to that time he took as placebos to please the patient, as symbols to reinforce words of "cheer and comfort." Of earlier physicians he said, approvingly: "Their learning was a learning in how to deal with men. Their skill was a skill in dealing with the emotions of men. They themselves were the therapeutic agents by which cures were effected. . . . The history of medicine is a history of the dynamic power of the relationship between doctor and patient."

Houston suggested a closer liaison between psychiatry and medicine, but he saw the relationship between the "neurotic" patient and the physician almost as an adversary one: "As the patient faces the doctor he believes in certain things about himself which the doctor doesn't believe. The patient has faith in his malady which the doctor doesn't share. . . . [the doctor] will prevail if his faith is stronger than the patient's faith." Given in such a mood, the placebo could become a challenge, not a gift, and might not mobilize helpful emotions, probably not what Houston had in mind. Of course a challenge to the right patient might prove very helpful in unmasking secondary gain, but challenging the patient with a placebo is not the way to go about it. For Houston the psychobiologic implications of disease were important. He wanted to strengthen the physician's faith in himself and, in his paternalistic times, saw the patient as the passive clay which the

20. Houston, W. R., The doctor himself as a therapeutic agent, *Ann. Intern. Med.* 11:1416–25, 1938.

physician could mold: "The faith that heals must have deep roots in the personality of the healer." Houston did not come to a firm conclusion, but he asked, "How can the doctor himself, as a therapeutic agent, be refined and polished to make of him a more potent agent?" That question is one that still needs to be asked today even if we may believe that the charismatic healing by the physician for which he was pleading is only one part of the drama. Certainly Houston can be counted among the first of those modern physicians who were calling for an understanding that not all of medical practice deals with the quantifiable: "One cannot advance against the disorders in the emotional sphere by mere reasoning."

Not too long ago a physician received a telephone call from a friend in another city, who told him that he had had a heart attack. "I am better now, but my doctor has offered me various alternative forms of therapy. I am very confused and I need your advice, even though you are a gastroenterologist." Advice duly given, he said, "You know, that is why I called. I know you don't know a damned thing about the heart, but I knew you would have an opinion, would state it directly and forcefully, and that makes me feel much better." As we will see, Franz Ingelfinger had similar comments about his own dilemma when he was asked to choose what treatment he should receive as a patient.[21] Thinking about the placebo should make us recall the relief that comes to most people when a physician says that we are in good shape.

Part of the charismatic talent must lie in the merging of the physician and the patient. As Burt puts it: "Many doctors and patients do clearly conceive themselves as psychologically merged in their dealings. . . . The patient's pain will vanish when he conceives himself and the world as one."[22]

In ideal circumstances the intent of the physician, the frame of mind in which he gives the placebo, might even be seen as a joining with the patient in a confession of ignorance that we do not always know how healing comes about, but we do know the force of the good patient-physician relationship. Transference and countertransference must be important in this regard, and are discussed in chapter 12.

As medical practice grows more rationally scientific, enlarging its already vast array of technical devices, of which the artificial heart is the latest example, and transplantation of brain tissue the newest dream, as medical science becomes more capable of treating organic disease, physicians are less and less able to come to terms with complaints which have no objective counterpart. Practitioners are criti-

21. Ingelfinger, F. J., Arrogance, *NEJM* 303:1507–11, 1980.
22. Burt, *Taking care of strangers.*

cized for being too cold and too uninterested because the techniques they understand the best and are the most comfortable with are those which involve technology. They are criticized for growing too rich from the rewards they receive for the use of that technology, a reproof which may be receding under the barrage of new cost-control measures.

Dangers for the Physician

There are perils for the physician in giving placebos because of their undoubted effectiveness. Because the placebo works, he may delude himself into thinking that the patient has no important organic disease. He may find the placebo the first step to more major forms of deceit or simply the road to a diagnostic and therapeutic ennui it would be hard to defend. In the worst instance the physician may use the response to a placebo as an indication that the disease or the complaint is feigned. The danger that he will overlook an organic disease, however, seems overemphasized even if the suffering from a cancer of the pancreas can be as great as from any existential pain, and sometimes as impressively assuaged.[23]

Finally we have to consider what may be the greatest danger of all for the physician, that giving a placebo will give him an even higher opinion of his own abilities to help. I do not wish to see physicians return to their former arrogant estimates of themselves, and giving a placebo as a magic potion without thinking about what he is doing might dangerously enhance the physician's self-image.

23. Bok, S., The ethics of giving placebos, *Scientific American* 231:17–22, 1974.

4

The Inert Pill

Most definitions, ignoring the intent of the physician, focus on the activity of the pill, on what is already known or measurable about a drug. A pill may have known or unknown activity. Objective data is what counts, but the problem comes in how to define *objective*. What is believed to be known at one time may turn out to be wrong later. What is "known" may prove only a half-truth, or less.

When we talk about a pill or a placebo, we have to remember that there are known, already discerned actions, and there are also unknown, as yet undetected actions. Grunbaum uses the term *characteristic* to refer to aspects of treatment that are known, and that fit into a therapeutic theory, and *incidental* to refer to those factors in a therapy which are unknown or simply considered side effects.[1]

Truth in medicine has moved from what the patient says to what the physician finds. Milk in the treatment of the pain of peptic ulcer offers a good example of the problems that come as objective data has replaced subjective reports, as only what is measurable is acceptable.[2] For many years milk was the staple of the ulcer diet, relieving dyspepsia and pain. The Sippy diets based on varying proportions of milk and cream were a standby in the management of peptic ulcer for many years, to most physicians' and patients' satisfaction. The cream was eliminated in the 1940s and 1950s because people taking it got too fat and doctors began to worry that too much cream in the diet might lead to heart attacks. Still, skimmed milk remained the mainstay of the program.

1. Grunbaum, A., The placebo concept, *Behav. Res. Therapy* 19:157–67, 1981.
2. Spiro, H. M., Is milk so bad for the peptic ulcer patient? *J. Clin. Gastroenterol.* 3:219–20, 1981.

Then, in the 1970s, laboratory studies suggested that milk could not neutralize gastric acid and—worse—could increase the amount of acid in the stomach. Physicians began advising their patients with peptic ulcer not to take milk because it might be making them worse, and instead gave them large amounts of antacids. The antacids had proven effective in neutralizing acid in the laboratory, and in experimental subjects, and therefore it seemed that such well-defined chemicals ought to be better than milk for people with duodenal ulcer. To be sure very few physicians could ever recall seeing a patient whose heartburn or indigestion worsened on drinking milk, but because it looked bad by laboratory evidence, milk was very quickly abandoned as serious therapy for the ulcer patient. Today the doctor who tells his patient to drink milk is thought to be invincibly ignorant.

More recent studies of exorphins[3] and prostaglandins have led to measurements which support the clinical reports that milk could indeed relieve peptic ulcer pain. Fascinating experiments have shown that milk and other foods, digested by pepsin-hydrochloric acid mixtures, have endorphin-like activity in experimental conditions.[4] Milk is digested to amino acids and polypeptides which in turn fill in endorphin receptors. Moreover it turns out that the phospholipids of milk are surface-protecting agents.[5] Again the details are not important, but it may well turn out over the next few years that milk will regain a place as a symptom reliever. My point is not to defend milk or dietary therapy, but simply to show how the reports of pain relief by patients are disparaged as "subjective" evidence which does not stand up, in physicians' minds at least, to the more "objective" evidence of the laboratory. Partial evidence, if quantified, seems better to most professionals than subjective reports. That is a problem in deciding what we mean by inactive or inert.

To call a substance inert is to say that it has no detectable physiologic or pharmacological effect. For the physician-scientist an inert substance is something which makes no measurable, detectable, *visible* change in what his instruments can measure. That it makes a change in what the patient reports is of no matter. Yet if I give an inert pill to a patient in pain and he is relieved, something has happened. How does an inert pill relieve pain? If a placebo relieves pain, can I claim that, in fact, it has an effect? Is it inert in these circumstances? Finally, if the physician has found a placebo to relieve pain before, can the knowledge that it has done so serve as a physiological or pharmaco-

3. Ibid.

4. Chang, K., Killian, A., Hazom, E., et al., Morphiception, *Science* 212:75–77, 1981.

5. Dial, E. J., and Lichtenberger, L. M., A role for milk phospholipids in protection against gastric acid, *Gastroenterology* 87:379–85, 1984.

logical prediction of clinical benefit? Can that experience be called knowledge? I think the physician can then say, "This pill has helped others and I hope therefore that it will help you, even if I don't understand how it works."

It is important to keep in mind that there are two kinds of inert pills: the pure and the impure placebo.

The *pure placebo* is, so far as is known, completely inert, being composed of a material such as starch or sugar; such a pill is given only for the patient's benefit. By this definition we usually mean that the substance given has no measurable effect in a laboratory beaker, so to speak, and that it has no detectable effect in a biological preparation, in a rat or dog or in any organ of such animal. The symbolic effect that the medicine might have to a human being, or the physiological effects of that symbolic effect are not taken into consideration except by a few behavioral scientists. Moreover, the problem is that what is deemed inactive at one time may prove to have physiologic effects later. Lactose pills, so beloved as inactive by an earlier generation, and a favorite placebo for investigators, turn out to have side effects of their own.

The *impure placebo* is a pill or drug with some pharmacological activity which is not immediately or seriously relevant to the clinical problem being treated. In a sense the impure placebo is given to help the patient, but an active agent is chosen for the benefit of the physician, to buttress his regard for himself as giving only active medications. Its action is inappropriate to the disease being treated. In this second category fall a vast array of sometimes harmless but active agents or injections which physicians give, usually knowingly, to convince themselves that they are giving a drug of some merit: the mild anticholinergic agents, multivitamins, antibiotics, and many other substances, cimetidine among them. Such drugs are active enough, with demonstrable pharmacologic consequences, so that the physician can console himself with the idea that the drug might work, even if he is not sure that the effect is aimed at the symptom that he is treating.

In supporting the role of physician therapy, what he calls "iatrotherapy", Feinstein comes down in favor of the impure placebo when he says: "If nothing else is available, a doctor who believes he has nothing to prescribe may be unwilling to prescribe a placebo and may thereby also eliminate himself as a therapeutic agent. . . . A safe pharmaceutical agent, with a reasonable rationale for usage, may sometimes be desirable even if some of its results are not substantially better than those of placebo."[6] That could be a definition of an over-

6. Feinstein, A. R., Should placebo-controlled trials be abolished? *Eur. J. Clin. Pharmac.* 17:1–4, 1980.

the-counter (OTC) drug, its effect augmented by the suggestion of advertising.

Moreover, if the pill has a side effect such as the dry mouth produced by anticholinergic drugs, the placebo effect may be enhanced, the patient surmising that if the drug is strong enough to dry his mouth, it must be doing some good elsewhere. From such considerations, I assume, came all the bitter tonics and pretty pills of the old pharmacopoeia. In general I agree with the idea that impure placebos do more harm than good. Whether in our malpractice-prone times an active placebo will prove stronger defense against a lawsuit than an inactive one is a matter for conjecture.

To some extent OTC drugs must have a large placebo effect given the context in which they are taken, the persuasive advertising that encourages their use, and the expectations that they will work. The FDA has been reviewing the effectiveness of so-called OTC drugs over the past decade and has winnowed many of them out of the market. The ones that are left have been thoroughly reviewed and have been deemed "safe and effective," in Category I. The difficulties inherent in comparing many of these drugs with placebo therapy, given the circumstances in which OTC drugs are taken, rather suggests that they represent a unique and certainly harmless (if directions are followed) combination of active drugs[7] whose effect is augmented by advertising, custom, and expectation.[8]

Extending the definition in chapter 2, I define a placebo as a medicine, pill, or liquid which is given by a physician in the belief that it is inactive and with the intent of relieving the symptom or making the patient feel better in some way. Medicines believed to be active and which later prove to be ineffective and to have worked only by virtue of their unforeseen placebo effect do not fall under this definition. The benefit of such an inactive medicine provides evidence for the placebo effect and enhances our belief in that effect, but such medicines are not being given as placebos in physician-patient communication. Obviously, therefore, operations are unlikely to be placebo in intent even though many operations have only a placebo effect, however much those who carry them out may believe otherwise. Less drastic interventions, such as gastrointestinal endoscopy, carried out to reassure the patient, can more seriously be considered to be placebo in intent. The doctor often feels that if he carries out a procedure which he expects to give normal results, the patient will be reassured. That, too, is hard to define as a placebo. Reassurance is not the

7. Pisani, J. M., Are over-the-counter drugs really placebos? Definitely not, in *Controversies in Therapeutics*, ed. L. Lasagna, Philadelphia: Saunders, 1980, pp. 33–40.

8. Jones, J. K., Do over-the-counter drugs act mainly as placebos? Yes, in *Controversies in Therapeutics*, ed. L. Lasagna, Philadelphia: Saunders, 1980, pp. 26–32.

same as suggestion or persuasion, though it would take more of a philosopher than I to evaluate the differences. Many procedures have a placebic effect but are not, strictly speaking, placebos.

PROCEDURES AS PLACEBO

Does a placebo have to be a pill, or can an injection, an operation, any procedure, even a simple diagnostic one, work as a placebo? Today diagnostic procedures so lavishly paid for by the Blue Shield plans are themselves so endowed with enthusiasm on the part of the physician and patient that they may be placebos, and are indeed so credited by many physicians. They may claim that the procedure is being done to reassure, yet the effect is that of a placebo.

Injection as Placebo

If there is any place where behavioral responses might prove to be important, it surely must be in the placebo response to injection. The act is definable, not conventional in the way that taking a pill is ordinary, and it requires the active intervention of someone else, nurse or physician. Giving an injection must be loaded with behavioral effects. Certainly there is much room for study of how often subjects have received injections before, for what reasons, and with what previous effect. It is possible that someone has examined whether the previous experience of the patient has anything to do with the benefit he receives from the injection. Most physicians have the impression a placebo given by injection is even more beneficial than one taken by mouth, but apparently the reasons for this have not been explored. B-12 injections are commonly given as a placebo, but there is little discussion of how, why, or whether a placebo is more effective as an injection than as a pill. Surely the symbol of something penetrating the body, being injected into it, must evoke stronger physiologic mechanisms, whatever they may be, than simply taking a pill, however sacramental the act of taking a pill may seem.

Lipkin long ago described using an iontophoresis apparatus as a placebo.[9] At the time the technique was thought to be helpful in patients with Raynaud's syndrome. Lipkin did not turn on the current, "but simply clicked the dials. Some improvement was reported in every case, and the results were excellent in six cases. Suggestion was undoubtedly responsible for the result in these."

9. Lipkin, M., McDevitt, E., Schwartz, S., et al., On the effects of suggestion in the treatment of vasospastic disorders of the extremities, *Psychosom. Med.* 7:152–57, 1945.

Operation as Placebo

Henry Beecher first emphasized that surgery could evoke a placebo effect and cautioned against interpreting the benefit of new operations until tests could be properly designed "to rule out the bias of the patient or the surgeon."[10] He pointed out the short cycle of two years, from enthusiasm to discredit, of the treatment of angina pectoris by mammary artery ligation.

Cardiovascular operations. In a wide-ranging multicenter study to evaluate coronary artery surgery, published in 1983, bypass operations relieved pain in a substantially larger number of patients than did medical treatment, but in other respects the results of medical treatment were just as good as those of surgery.[11] People who had only medical therapy lived just as long as those who had undergone operation, and they were just as likely to return to work. In other words the main detectable benefit of cardiac surgery seemed to be relief of pain, at least in this study. Asked why this should be most cardiologists usually ascribe pain relief after operation to interruption of pain fibers by the surgery, or to a more profuse growth of blood vessels into the heart muscle as a result of the inflammation brought about by the operation, and then suggest that such relief of ischemia is the important factor. Not many of them are willing to accept the suggestion that the operation might also have a placebo benefit. Yet just looking at the very impressive scar on your chest, knowing that a surgeon has had your heart in his hands and that an operation to improve the blood supply has been carried out, surely must give some push to faith if not to endorphin levels.[12] The symbol of that scar over the heart must be important even if unexamined, and a constant source of relief. One hundred sixty thousand of such operations were done in 1982, and in 1984 the number had risen to over two hundred thousand, with a mortality rate of 3 percent.

Gastrointestinal operations. Skeptics have long noted that an operation, particularly a new one, seems to bring benefit for several years until it is reevaluated and then often abandoned. This is particularly true of operations designed to relieve abdominal pain. The process is often tied up with the discovery of a new syndrome by a new technological diagnostic device. Findings by such a new device are wrenched

10. Beecher, H. K., Surgery as placebo, *JAMA* 176:1102–07, 1961.
11. CASS principle investigators: Coronary Artery Surgery Study (CASS), A randomized trial of coronary artery bypass surgery, *Circulation* 68:939–50, 1983.
12. Moerman, D. E., Anthropology of symbolic healing, *Current Anthropol.* 20:59–80, 1979.

into place as an explanation for abdominal pain, then advanced as a universal explanation. Attempts are made to eradicate the effects by operation or by drugs, and only after some years is it clear that the original finding was not as important as it had seemed nor were the operations successful for very long. In my own field of gastroenterology many explanations for abdominal pain have been advanced over the past thirty years, although, so far as I know, neither the diagnostic procedure nor the operation designed to remove what it has uncovered has been credited with a placebo effect.

A good, if hardy, example is offered by the woman with abdominal pain of uncertain cause, a common and challenging phenomenon to practitioners' offices. In the 1950s, as radiologic studies of the stomach became more sophisticated and fluoroscopic techniques improved, antral pyloric mucosal prolapse was detected on fluoroscopy. Found in young women with abdominal pain (because there were more of them coming to be X-rayed) it was deemed the cause of abdominal pain, nausea, and belching. Once a lesion is found there is an irresistible temptation to remove it or fix it, and so at least several hundred women underwent operations to remove the bottom part of the stomach or to tighten up the pyloric prolapse. The operation proved worthless after a few years and was abandoned.

A few years later angiographic techniques to visualize the vessels of the body came into vogue as a valuable diagnostic approach. Angiography led to the detection of so-called celiac axis stenosis in women with abdominal pain, which was touted as a cause of the pain. After quite a few blood vessels had been loosened up at operation with only short-term benefit, the concept was abandoned.

More recently radioactive techniques have made it possible to measure the rapidity with which the stomach empties itself of food. As might have been expected some stomachs empty faster than others. Now the same kind of women who a few years ago stood accused of celiac axis stenosis or antral mucosal prolapse are told that they have delayed gastric emptying. Such women take drugs to speed up the sluggish emptying, and if that does not work they run the risk of a drainage procedure to promote emptying. As this series of observations are still relatively new and the enthusiasm of my colleagues remains correspondingly high, I cannot yet conclude that the process is just another in a long series of ill-conceived notions. I suspect that it will prove to be no more effective than operations in the 1920s to tie down a "floating" kidney or restoring to its resting place a "mobile" cecum.

Sham operations. In the 1980s it would be deemed unethical, even with informed consent, to carry out a sham operation designed to simulate an operation to be evaluated. Yet in the 1950s two groups of surgeons carried out just such a double-blind trial of internal mammary artery ligation.[13] That operation was believed to increase blood flow through the coronary arteries by stimulating collateral circulation. In their trials these groups incised the skin under local anesthesia in all patients, but ligated the internal mammary artery in only half of them. The results were surprising at the time: *All* the patients who had undergone sham ligation reported a decreased need for nitroglycerin and increased exercise tolerance; only 76 percent of the patients whose mammary artery had actually been tied reported the same improvement. Over all at least 49 percent of all patients reported improvement, ligation of the internal mammary artery giving no more relief than a simple skin incision.

Later, implantation of the internal mammary artery into a tunnel in the myocardium, the so-called Vineberg operation, in the hope that a collateral circulation would develop between the artery and the coronary blood vessels became popular. An improvement rate of 85 percent was reported, but as improvement never correlated with objective angiographic evidence, the procedure was finally abandoned in part because coronary artery bypass surgery had been developed. Nevertheless, Benson points out, "Before the procedure was abandoned, 10,000 to 15,000 operations were performed, with an average operative mortality of approximately 5%."[14] In these studies, the reviewers conclude, "In addition to subjective improvement, objective changes occurred: The placebo effect increased exercise tolerance, reduced nitroglycerin usage, and improved electrocardiographic results. . . . Patient and physician belief in the efficacy of the therapy and a continuously strong physician-patient relationship should maintain the effects for long periods." A believer in the placebo effect, Benson comments, "This remarkable efficacy should not be disregarded or ridiculed. After all, unlike most other forms of therapy, the placebo effect has withstood the test of time and continues to be safe and inexpensive." He emphasized the importance of communicating confidence in the therapy, but unlike most commentators when confronted with the criticism that it might be deceptive to appear more confident than can be justified by the evidence, still calls for "reasonable enthusiasm to increase the placebo effect by such confidence."

13. Cobb, L. A., Thomas, G. I., Dillard, D. H., et al., An evaluation of internal-mammary-artery ligation by a double-blind technique, *NEJM* 260:1115–18, 1959; Dimond, E. G., Kittle, C. F., and Crockett, J. E., Comparison of internal mammary ligation and sham operation for angina pectoris, *Am. J. Cardiol.* 5:483–86, 1960.

14. Benson, H., and McCallie, D. P., Angina pectoris and the placebo effect, *NEJM* 300:1424–29, 1979.

The fascinating point, of course, is why such operations help patients for even a short while. Changed perception, attention deviated to the pain of the operation, the care that the patient receives, the attending mystery of the operation itself, and finally, the symbolic value of the scar on chest or belly might all contribute. The history of modern medicine is replete with such examples which should be embarrassing to us all. Conceivably operations work as placebos because of the enormous metabolic changes that they engender: sooner or later, when endorphins and enkephalins and cholecystokinins, or some other hormones, can be measured, there will doubtless prove to be considerable change in their levels and only then will we physicians begin to recognize that such operations are indeed arduous placebos.

Bouginage as Placebo

Many procedures act as placebos. One recent study is illuminating. Bouginage of the esophagus is said to relieve the chest pain of patients with esophageal spasm, and most gastroenterologists treat such patients by passing a large bougie into the esophagus in the belief that stretching it makes it incapable of quite such fierce contractions. Some Navy physicians, therefore, studied the response of eight patients over a period of sixteen weeks to "placebo" bouginage.[15] As placebo or control they passed a small bougie, 24F in diameter, because a dilator of that narrow caliber is believed too thin to stretch the esophagus. The patients receiving "treatment" underwent dilation with a 54F bougie "because of its real therapeutic potential." At the end of sixteen weeks there proved to be no difference between the effects of the small or large bougie, either on the degree or frequency of chest pain or, surprisingly enough, on the frequency or degree of dysphagia. The authors concluded that there was a significant decrease in the severity of chest pain in *all* patients regardless of the size of the dilator simply over the course of the observations and, we can assume, because of the attention that the patients received: "It is our impression that one possible mechanism might be a placebo-like effect arising from the close physician-patient interaction in this study. . . . In the setting of a close physician-patient interaction the patient appears to respond to intervention."

15. Winters, C., Artnak, E. J., Benjamin, S. B., et al., Esophageal bouginage in symptomatic patients with the nutcracker esophagus, *JAMA* 252:363–66, 1984.

5

The Patient and His Disease: Pharmacology and Faith

The patient who receives the placebo plays the leading role in the placebo drama. His expectations about the pill or procedure, his reaction to his disease and his doctor, his outlook on life, will all prove important to the placebo effect. People respond to a medicine because of its pharmacological effect or because they have faith in it and in the doctor, or because of both. Patients may not respond to a pill or procedure because they have no faith in it, or in their doctor. The patient is as important as the disease. The discussion to follow in the next few chapters will touch on the relation between the patient and his physician, particularly in relation to the popular topics of patient equality and autonomy or self-determination. Ideas on these matters have changed what physicians do to their patients, or at least how they talk about what needs to be done.

I sometimes think that the teaching function of the doctor has usurped his old-fashioned benevolent caring role. Some current doctors are more interested in telling the truth than in helping their patients get well. I find myself wondering whether always telling the truth does more to buttress the doctor's good opinion of his own uprightness than it does to help the patient in his calamity. Some doctors insist on telling the truth more to have a higher respect for their own integrity than to help their patients. Such a view may sound paternalistic, but I am sure that the fatherly role is not always a bad one, or that the patient in need of help is not equally in need of some advice along with paternal (or maternal) reassurance. It may even be that unconscious, or even collective, guilt at being able to do so little for patients makes physicians all the more insistent on telling the truth. Some academic discussions of patient equality lack the ring of truth to me and pay too little attention to the distant protests of the practicing physician. How can we physicians give patients relief *and* knowledge? These are the questions that will occupy us now.

WHAT IS A PATIENT?

What is a patient? There is little formal discussion in medical papers on placebo, or anywhere else for that matter, about what a patient is. *Webster's* accepts a patient as "one that suffers, endures, or is victimized" and notes that this is an archaic definition, but we could see it as one that proponents of the inherently adversarial relationship between physician and patient might adopt. The more workable second definition describes a patient as "a sick individual, especially when awaiting or under the care and treatment of a physician or surgeon." The *OED* defines a patient as "a sufferer. . . . one who is under medical treatment . . . a person or thing that undergoes some reaction." The incorporation of "suffering" in patienthood is now old-fashioned, probably reflecting the transitions of medicine from the subjective to the objective.

Patient Role and Sick Role

Sociologists are careful to separate the patient role from the sick role, a distinction which has some bearing on the placebo.[1] Someone may be sick but yet not see himself as a patient. He becomes a patient when he looks for help. To become a patient is to encounter a healer in the expectation that the latter will do something to alleviate or change what is affecting the sick person. Many observers see the ensuing encounter as a reality negotiation, a situation in which patient and physician are grappling. The metaphor, reminiscent of Buber, seems appropriate for what goes on. The patient needs to give an account of the problem or complaint, a description of symptoms. Then, after the physician has formed an impression, the symptoms might be reinterpreted and the account rephrased. What is usually a mundane meeting for a physician turns out for the patient to be an exceptional, expensive, and often alarming encounter, which may or may not end in reassurance. The encounter is inherently unequal: the patient seeks help, knows less than the physician about what is wrong with him in the technical sense, and comes full of anxiety and foreboding, or at least incommoded.

1. Twaddle, A. C., Sickness and the sickness career: Some implications, in *The relevance of social science for medicine*, ed. L. Eisenberg and A. Kleinman, Dordrecht: Reidel, 1981, pp. 111–33.

In recent times physicians' notions about patients have changed. The old concept of the ideal patient as passive, compliant, and dependent on the physician who is captain of the ship has yielded to the ideal of the patient as an equal partner with the physician, equal except in specific knowledge. Of course patients come in more varieties than physicians, even if in what follows I discuss "the" patient. Each will have a different idea not only of what being sick means, but also, possibly, a different model of what he expects his physician to be. Nowadays physicians are more accustomed to thinking of equality in the patient-physician relationship. The older ones, as I have already suggested, would like to go back to being captain of the ship, a metaphor that can be traced to Plato. Their concept of equality implies that the doctor has moved off his pedestal, not that the patient has come up to the doctor's level. Very few physicians born since the 1930s see themselves as servants of their patients. Yet some patients must see the doctor as very little different from the tailor, the furniture polisher, or the teacher, essential but hired to do a specific job and no more. Not everyone wants to be prodded and pushed in every area of life and health by the physician.

The patient's previous history affects not only his response to placebos, but his notion of how close he wants the therapeutic alliance to be, and of what kind. Family, environment, nurture, and many other social factors impossible to cover in this brief account go into making up a personality, and they all will influence what a patient wants. I will conclude later that everyone can be a placebo responder, but even though I treat patients as a generic patient in this account, I do not consider issues of personality and past history, experiences not only with other doctors but with other people, unimportant. Byck emphasizes how the patient's expectations of what a drug can do influences not only his concept of how the drug works and how other drugs work, but to a large extent may even influence his response to a placebo.[2] To write more of these matters would be to write another book.

Patients and Cases

The difference between a patient and a case is what it is all about. The *patient* is the person who has the disease. The *case* is the record of the course of the disease in a person. The emphasis in the case is upon the disease as an entity; it tells of the life of the disease, not the life of the patient.

2. Byck, R., Psychologic factors in drug administration, in *Clinical Pharmacology*, eds. K. Melman and H. Morelli, New York: Macmillan, 1978.

Yet the physician who looks only at the physical factors, at the case, the medical student who is taught to concentrate simply on the strict biomedical level, will miss most of illness. Fabrega puts it well:

> One who reduces medical problems to physical factors concentrates on genes, biochemistry, physiology, and disease entities and examines how these are affected by the culture-nature interaction which prevails in the society at question. Symbolizations about personal concerns, including those of illness, are likely to be judged as incidental "surface phenomena" far removed from the substantive aspects of disease. . . . A limitation of the reductionist's program, however, is that suffering, functioning, and level and quality of adaptation are excluded. . . . In contrast to the above, one who emphasizes the interconnections between biological, psychological, and social factors will judge individuals holistically, resist body-mind partitioning, and describe a medical problem or illness as something rooted in and expressed by social adaptation and function.[3]

Part of the problem in dealing with the relief of pain comes in the differing models of disease that physician and patient have. Trained to see himself as a scientist, even if a recent immigrant from the country of faith healers, the modern physician yearns for organic disease, wants to make a diagnosis. Most patients, I think, are concerned as much with what they feel, with getting relief, with getting rid of their pain as anything else. They are also worried about the prognosis: "Is this serious?" Physicians are trained in medical school and residency in the detection of structural defects. Nowhere in training is there much time for considering the unspoken and the unseen. If in practice patients come to doctors with existential pain for which there is no apparent physical basis, the physician will not rest until he has gone through all the diagnostic studies.

Many patients, of course, come with the same expectations, and even if told that a given test has a one in a hundred chance of detecting an abnormality, they will often choose to undergo it, to be sure. Health economists should perhaps examine patient expectations as closely as the habits of physicians. Even in a theoretical discussion the most intelligent lay colleagues want a pain followed down as carefully and closely as possible, in order to find its cause, rather than simply accept relief of the pain. This shows an excessive faith in what physicians can do.

3. Fabrega, H., The idea of medicalization: An anthropological perspective, *Perspectives Biol. Med.* 24:129–42, 1980.

Effect of Placebo on Patients

Patients are relieved of pain and comforted by placebos, often enough so that the observer might expect something good to be said of them. But in the 1980s that is very rarely the case.

Most arguments against the placebo from the patient's standpoint seem to involve one or more of the following: (1) self-determination (comments involve being lied to, being deceived); (2) economics (arguments revolve around paying for useless drugs); (3) education (being trained to think that doctors are all-powerful and that pills are necessary for every disorder); and (4) diagnostic delay (some observers, more naive than others, believe that any pill or placebo will delay the appropriate diagnostic events and that the patient will therefore fare badly.)

In the next chapter we examine what kinds of patients with what kinds of diseases or illnesses respond to placebo in a predictable enough way to evaluate. For now it will simplify matters if we consider the placebo given in good faith—what I have called a gift—rather than the range of placebo giving.

The Placebo Effect: Report and Response

"Many papers have demonstrated the importance and magnitude of the placebo effect in every therapeutic area. Placebos can be more powerful than, and reverse the action of, potent active drugs. The incidence of placebo reactions approaches 100% in some studies. Placebos can have profound effects on organic illnesses, including incurable malignancies. Placebos can often mimic the effects of active drugs."[4] Although Shapiro's comment has been widely quoted, it is hard from the vantage point of the 1980s to substantiate his wide generalizations. His summary did not distinguish firmly the difference between reports of a patient's response to the placebo and improvement in the disease itself. Yet his observation has been reiterated with remarkable fidelity by most commentators, especially those who are not physicians, as accurately reflecting the power of placebos, and it has had an enormous influence on subsequent discussions. But most of the original material, reviewed in the next chapter, is less convincing. Whatever the placebo does, the nature of the response has been obscured by uncritical, even rapturous claims. The placebo benefit depends on one person's responding to another. The person is helped, but the disease goes unchanged except insofar as the natural healing processes (whatever they may prove to be) are engaged. Subjective complaints are relieved, to a greater or lesser extent, but there exists

4. Shapiro, A. K., The placebo response, in *Modern perspectives in world psychiatry*, ed. J. G. Howells, Edinburgh: Oliver and Boyd, 1968.

no convincing evidence that diseases are changed, for better or worse. That is not to deny that people can die of fright, of voodoo, hexing, or even of anxiety. Such matters are well documented, and in the medical world are ascribed to heart irregularities, electrolyte imbalance, and other functional disequilibriums.[5] Evidence is simply lacking that structural improvement has come about from the direct effect of a placebo.

DISEASE AND ILLNESS

First we have to try to distinguish between disease and the reaction to it. If I hit my thumb with a hammer, my thumb hurts. The pain is in my thumb, but if it is bad enough I may hop around on one foot yelling, "Oh, oh!" My reaction to the pain may prove more impressive than the injury to my thumb. The middle-aged man who develops a new pain in his stomach may ignore it, take some antacid, or worry that he has a cancer. If the pain goes away on its own, he will be relieved, but may watch what he eats for a while. If it persists, he will grow more worried until anxiety, more than pain, drives him to the doctor. He may begin to feel better just deciding to see a physician. Every physician has had patients say, "You know, Doctor, ever since I made the appointment, I have felt well. I don't know why I'm here, but I thought I should come anyway." Relief may have been spontaneous, for which the physician's secretary or the telephone company could claim equal credit, but it could be related to the connection established with the physician. Of course, one can argue, as I do, that most sickness goes away on its own, and that the patient may have made the appointment when he felt the worst, just before the trouble began to wane. Because of such natural waxing and waning of disease, such anecdotal experience is hard to solidify, but it may not be any less real.

Is such pain then solely from the stomach? If you see your doctor for indigestion and, after examination, he says that you are fine, you may feel better and your pains may go away because of such reassurance, regardless of what medication you take. If, on the other hand, he looks grave and orders X-rays or even endoscopy, you will surely feel worse, or at least you will be more attentive to the pain. If, without a smile, the physician says, "Take this prescription for ten days, but be careful, because it has side effects," you may worry even more.

5. Engel, G. L., Psychologic stress, vasodepressor (vasovagal) syncope, and sudden death, *Ann. Intern. Med.* 89:403–12, 1978; Lex, B. W., Voodoo death: New thoughts on an old explanation, *Amer. Anthropologist* 76:818–22, 1974.

You may be uncertain as to whether it is hope that makes you better —or the pill, or anxiety that makes you worse—or the feared cancer! The important point is that the disease and the patient form one part of an equation of which the physician makes up another part.

Physicians do not all agree on what they mean by *disease*. For most the *OED* will suffice: "a condition of the body, or some part or organ of the body, in which its functions are disturbed or deranged; a morbid physical condition; . . . a departure from the state of health especially when caused by structural change." *Disorder* on the other hand, is defined as: "a disturbance of the bodily or mental functions; . . . usually a weaker term than disease, and not implying structural change." There are obvious problems with these definitions; disordered function must reflect structural change, which may be at the level of the twists and turns of amino acids or even, finally, of electrical forces. But the practicing physician is a pragmatist. He defines disease as something he can detect morphologically, biochemically, or simply functionally. The philosophical, medical, and legal literature is replete with definitions of disease, all of which involve a value judgment. Here I will use the term as it is generally understood by physicians: that which the clinician can detect by his instruments, and most of all by his eyes, in a person who has a complaint. In short, the term *disease* is used here to mean an abnormality which is *biologically detectable* and which shows up on the physician's screens or panels, whether these are represented as images or numbers.[6]

Organic and Functional Disease

Organic disease. By organic modern physicians mean something which is anatomically or biomedically detectable, preferably with morphological reflections. That is why modern genetics is so entrancing: we see form and function at their most elemental. DNA makes the code, RNA transmits it, but change the direction of an amino acid and the message and the person are changed as well. It is no accident that the genetic code is metaphorically an alphabet: a d.o.g. is not a g.o.d. The physician is happiest calling a disease something that he can see by X-ray or other imaging techniques, or by touch and feel—anything that has a biological origin. Seeing and touching are his favorite diagnostic senses, the eyes and the fingers his oldest diagnostic tools. Pneumonia displayed on the X-ray film, or an ulcer scrutinized endoscopically and photographed to show others, provide the forms of disease with which he is the most comfortable, although he has learned to recognize molecular perturbations as disease. His training

6. Spiro, H. M., The tools of our trade—some comments on disease and disorder, *NEJM* 292:575–78, 1975.

section. Here I want to emphasize their unreality for the physician trained as a scientist to look at data and as a clinician to gaze at images.

The irritable bowel. Many people have diarrhea, constipation, or characteristic abdominal pain for much of their lives, often at times of stress. Many of them accept such disordered bowel function as normal (which I think it is) and do not go to a doctor. Others look for medical help. Why do some seek help and others not? Anxiety must have something to do with it; in a North Carolina study people who went to their doctors about abdominal pain were more likely to ascribe it to stressful events than people with abdominal pain who did not seek out doctors.[15]

Usually the physician can recognize such an irritable bowel, particularly in a young person, just by listening to the story. But he very likely will not rest there, content with what the patient tells him. Instead he has been trained to carry out a host of studies, their number depending upon his degree of sophistication, to "prove" the diagnosis. For the irritable bowel recognized by symptoms, and even in its surrounding sociocultural matrix, remains vague until it is decorated with a special wave pattern which can be duly unrolled on a strip of paper and passed from hand to hand. To a large extent, I fear, many clinicians believe that the number of diseases which can be recognized only from symptoms, by the ear, will diminish as technology improves, as knowledge expands. Ultimately they suspect that new organizing principles, neurotransmitters maybe, will enable them to put all functional disease into a morphologic mold.

Illness

Illness is what is felt by the patient, regardless of whether he has a detectable disease.[16] It is important to distinguish what can be seen by the physician from what is felt by the patient. Leon Eisenberg put it flatly: "Patients suffer 'illnesses'; physicians diagnose and treat diseases."[17] Patients are sometimes loathe to intrude on this division. Lefton, a sociologist with Parkinsonism wrote, "I think of the many times I have left my doctor's office taking with me the non-medical trials and tribulations that are not his concern as a professional spe-

15. Sandler, R. S., Drossman, D. A., Nathan, H. D., et al., Symptom complaints and health care seeking behavior in subjects with bowel dysfunction, *Gastroenterol.* 87: 314–18, 1984.

16. Kleinman, A. S., Eisenberg, L., and Good, B., Culture, illness, and care: Clinical lessons from anthropologic and cross-cultural research, *Ann. Intern. Med.* 88:251–58, 1978.

17. Eisenberg, L., Disease and illness: Distinctions between professional and popular ideas of sickness, *Culture, Medicine, and Psychiatry* 1:9–23, 1977.

makes him happy to accept the notion that brain-events are mind-events. When he reads that calcium flux and changes in cyclic AMP account for memory in the mollusk, he expects that ultimately even human behavior will be reduced to biochemistry.[7] He does not ask the locus of hope or fear, or free will, but expects that all emotions will prove to be reducible to some searching process in the computer model of the brain. He applauds the idea that even grammar is innate, simply a specialized hardware that will some day be visible to the scientist. He would agree with Bouillaud: "If there is an axiom in medicine, it is certainly the proposition that there is no disease without a seat. If one accepted the contrary opinion, one would also have to admit that there existed functions without organs, which is a palpable absurdity."[8] He would disagree with Cavell, who said: "We don't know whether the mind is best represented by the phenomenon of pain, or by that of envy, or by working on a jigsaw puzzle, or by a ringing in the ears."[9]

In the past the body was seen as a machine and the mind, in Arthur Koestler's words, as "the ghost in the machine." Now mind-body problems are no longer very important, but the brain is seen as a computer running the body machine. There is no room for the ecstatic visionary idea, only reason and objectivity.

Scientists confidently expect that some day the brain will be mapped, each neuron traced to all of its connections, its computer network so well laid out that we will know the place of hope and love, of all our aspirations, and all our aspirations will turn out to be neurotransmitted programs. Depression offers a current example: once thought to be repressed anger, now it seems to be a catecholamine deficiency relieved by chemicals. If that is true of depression, they suggest, will it not some day be true also of heroism? In a one-millimeter worm, *C. elegans*, investigators have now reconstructed 1,000 serial section electron micrographs to display the detailed anatomy and connections of the 302 neurons which make up this creature's "brain".[10] Those 302 neurons divided into 118 types make 8,000 synapses throughout the worm's small body. But for the reductionist this is the first step toward understanding the mind.

The mind-brain dichotomy is so tantalizing and so bewildering. How easy it would be if thought was secreted by the brain like acid from the stomach. Is the brain a pancreas or a computer? On the

7. Kandell, E. R., Schwartz, S. H. Molecular biology of learning, *Science* 218: 433–43, 1982.

8. Foucault, M., *The birth of the clinic*, New York: Vintage, 1973, p. 140.

9. Cavell, S., *Must we mean what we say?* Cambridge: Cambridge University Press, 1976, p. 265.

10. Lewin, R., The continuing tale of a small worm, *Science* 225:153–56, 1984.

computer model some argue that even dreams can be traced to specific neuronal activity. Where once it was boasted that a few years would suffice to unravel the neural connections of the brain, now even so ardent a neurobiologist as Winson recognizes that a little more time will be required to understand what he calls the neuronal logic of the brain, "the way brain structures work in unison to produce psychological function and behavior."[11] Winson describes how the important processing areas lie in the neocortex dependent upon the so-called cortical column, a vertical structure of neurons running from the top to the bottom of the neocortex (about one-tenth of an inch). Each column contains about 110 neurons and each of the estimated 600 million columns in the neocortex responds to a particular angle line or shape. Winson estimates that there are 50 billion neurons in the neocortex alone. In the limbic system brain circuits "generate emotion, link emotion to perception, and provide an impetus to behavior." Winson is an optimist: "One hopes and expects that in the course of time, measured perhaps in tens of years, the way the brain handles information during waking and sleeping behavior will be revealed."

He is not alone in his optimism; Wagner, extolling the positron-emission tomography studies of the brain with radioactive tracer molecules, remarks: "We now have a new set of eyes that permit us to begin to examine the chemistry of the mind."[12]

Obviously physicians and scientists will begin to trace out some of the shifting mechanisms. For Winson the brain is hard-wired like a computer mainframe; emotions, external cirucmstances, and the like simply provide different programs to switch functioning circuits around. That metaphor would not have been possible before the computer had been invented, and newer scientific discoveries will lead us to newer models of the brain, possibly more complex, but possibly even simpler. Quantum physics with its acceptance of uncertainty should eventually provide a great stimulus to the understanding of the billions of brain neurons. Physicists have trouble going from a small unit to a large collection and, dealing with artificial intelligence, they build models that resemble what happens when a flock of birds swirls, all moving together, or a school of fish swims by, all turning together. Perhaps the brain is more like a school of fish than a computer and great new ideas are more like the sudden turns of a flock of birds than the lighting-up of circuits. Being less optimistic than the experts, I believe that while we will understand more of the brain's circuitry, we will not soon know the locus of thoughts and the

11. Winson, J., *Brain and psyche*, New York: Anchor Press/Doubleday, 1985.
12. Wagner, H. N., Probing the chemistry of the mind. *NEJM* 312:44–46, 1985.

place of our hopes. We may yet view the mechanisms of the brain, the content of its thoughts will require a voice, or a pen, to app Auden was no reductionist when he wrote:

> If all a top physicist knows
> About the Truth be true . . .
> We have a better time
> Then the Greater Nebulae do,
> Or the atoms in our brains.[13]

How the mind emerges from the brain is beyond me. I will tinue to regard the mind and brain as different, for my purp just as I use the illness/disease dichotomy, a little fearful of fu discoveries.

The triumph of antibiotics over many infectious diseases has vided the model for disease with which the practicing physici most comfortable. Metaphor is important in all aspects of life, an large extent the concept of disease as enemy, the physician as so or detective, dominates medical thinking. The training of physi has taught them to regard themselves as detectives of organic dis not as relievers of symptoms. They regard any deviation from strictly scientific objective approach almost as religious thinke gard sin. The physician's metaphor of disease as an alien invade the body keeps him from accepting the idea of disease as illne matter how many commentators urge him to. Yet only when we of disease as the interaction between the organic process and th tient's response will physicians begin to grasp how the placebo c helpful. We must separate the reaction to the disease from the d itself and, as we contemplate what the placebo does, keep in mir difference between the patient and his disease. More than that, shall see, the clinician needs to make himself think of illness as disease and to make his goal the relief of suffering.

Functional Disease

Clinical experience for 150 years has been, as Foucault ha gested, the "anatomo-clinical gaze."[14] Functional diseases, tho lections of complaints for which no structural derangement found as an explanation—illnesses really—have little reality physician. Most physicians prefer to take care of people with ganic diseases they have been trained to recognize. It is these tional diseases that we will call illness, as I will discuss in th

13. Auden, W. H., After reading a child's guide to modern physics, in *poems*, New York: Random House, 1976, p. 557.
14. Foucault, *The birth of a clinic*.

cialist. To worry about what I worry about could severly handicap his practice as a neurologist."[18]

The response of the person to a disease, what has been called the *illness*, is determined by character, culture, and many other aspects of the person. It is a composite of disease and how it affects the patient who has it and how the disease is regarded by his society.[19] For many illness includes all the undesirable concomitants of the disease—the effect on the family, on their grief, and on everything in daily life. In short, disease is the primary process and illness, for the most part, may be deemed secondary.

Attribution. What a person thinks has caused his trouble, what he attributes his disease to, is also important. I will ignore this area except to confirm my agreement that the patient's explanatory model needs to be explored with the patient by the physician. Sociologists use the term *attribution* to define what the patient thinks has caused his illness. To a large extent the individual's notions are likely to be a reflection of the larger group's ideas. In the 1980s exercise, nutrition, and other matters seem to be more important to the lay person than emotion or even stress in causing disease, but their meaning to physician and patient may not always be the same.

Of course, not every fanciful model of disease has a basis in reality. Many popular explanatory models may have been dead wrong, in all senses. Sontag reminds us that tuberculosis was romanticized as a disease of passion, as the ravages of frustration, before its cause was known. "Many of the literary and erotic attitudes known as 'romantic agony' derive from tuberculosis."[20]

Value judgments. There are value judgments associated with the definitions of illness. As Boorse puts it: "A disease is an illness only if it is serious enough to be incapacitating and therefore is 1) undesirable for its bearer; 2) a title to special treatment; and, 3) a valid excuse for normally criticizable behavior."[21] I would prefer the term *unwelcome* to *undesirable*, as the latter seems to put some of the value judgment outside the person with the disease.

18. Lefton, M., Chronic disease and applied sociology: An essay in personalized sociology, *Sociological Inquiry* 54:466–76, 1984.

19. Fabrega, H., A behavioral framework for the study of human disease, *Ann. Intern Med.* 84:200–08, 1976; Eisenberg, L., The subjective in medicine, *Persp. Biol. Med.* 27:48–61, 1983.

20. Sontag, S., *Illness as metaphor*, New York: Random House, 1979, p. 28.

21. Boorse, C., On the distinction between disease and illness, *Philosophy and Public Affairs* 5:49–68, 1975.

Self-image. Illness, of course, will itself depend on many other features: (1) The person's view of himself is important. The professional tennis player will have a different interpretation of pain in his elbow and shoulder from the lawyer. (2) The culture in which the patient finds himself plays, as Fabrega puts it, "a critical role in how illness is determined."[22] The effect of a disease on social adaptation, on one's place in society, and the like all have an important role in determining how serious an "illness" appears. The physician who looks at disease only on a reductionistic model will attend to biochemical and structural perturbations, but will ignore the social and cultural problems that contribute to the illness.[23] He even may be annoyed at having such factors called to his attention, whereas the physician who looks at illness as well as disease may feel the obligation to see the patient in a far wider context. That second physician may help the patient more, and he probably is likely to order fewer tests in pursuit of every complaint.

Everyday experience assures us that illness is more than just having something wrong with an organ. The young man with Meniere's disease may turn out to have scarring in his cochlear apparatus, but he is not dizzy all of the time. The man with ulcerative colitis may have a small scarred, shriveled colon which he can ignore three months out of four. Many factors make complaints come and go, rise or fall in importance. They may be as banal as the weather or as intimate as family or friends; they may have to do with work or play.

Placebo, disease, and illness. In discussing the placebo I will use the term *illness* to refer to the patient's complaints, regardless of whether they have a biologically detectable origin. I will not use the term *disorder* except as synonymous with disease, even though I think it strikes a useful minor chord. Illness, as I will use the term, may or may not originate in disease, but it is the *subjective* component. Disease may or may not eventuate in symptoms, but it stands for the quantifiable biologically detectable aspects, the daily stuff of medical practice.

The reason for insisting on this distinction lies in the attempt to evaluate what the placebo does. It is the response to the illness that my review suggests the placebo affects. Placebos help people, not diseases. Such a distinction is not clearly respected in the literature, where pain is treated as an entity—reified as the philosophers put it—and the distinctions between disease and illness are not honored. If pain goes away, many observers conclude that a disease has been helped.

22. Fabrega, The idea of medicalization.
23. Fabrega, A behavioral framework.

Many other factors, not all quantifiable, play a part in bringing symptoms to attention. But curiously, what a person's mind brings to his experience of a disease, whether foreboding or annoyance, is not often explicitly discussed by physicians or medical teachers. Discussions of peptic ulcer therapy, for example, focus on the proper dose and frequency of the H2 blocker and on the relative importance of aspirin, smoking, or alcohol. Little interest is shown in the emotional or social life of a patient. Yet any group of physicians will all nod in agreement when asked whether emotions are important in the recurrences of peptic ulcer. Why are such issues ignored in formal discussions? Partly because physicians can do so little about them, except to listen, but more because there is nothing to measure and because we can depict structural or biological perturbations so exactly. Partly too, I must admit, because the H2 blockers can speed the healing of ulcers even if the physician ignores the emotional aspects of his patient.

That is a major obstacle. We can talk to a patient with peptic ulcer very little differently from the way Osler might have, but if we relied only on Osler's medical treatments the lawyers will soon be at our door. Psychiatry may have given us new visions of why a man gets an ulcer, but science has given us the H2 blockers with which to treat him, and they are so effective that we think we no longer need to talk to the patient. Interest in the psychological factors in ulcerative colitis waned as soon as steroids made therapy briskly effective. Before 1950, recovery from colitis came about only slowly and with immense effort by physician and patient to understand his life and his illness, but no one was quite certain whether remission was the result of the "natural history of the disease" or more specifically came from the patient-physician relationship. Once steroids speeded up the healing process, the work of the physician became very much easier. Three to five days of intravenous ACTH effected a remission which before might have taken months. People with inflammatory bowel disease now get better very much quicker than before, but they know very much less about themselves than they once did, and their doctors seem glad to be rid of that burden. Such examples suggest that the patient's notion of what is wrong with him can be ignored, and the doctor's too for that matter, once an injection or a pill eliminates the problem.

The patient as a whole: Systems medicine. For a long time thoughtful physicians, often trained as psychiatrists or interested in the behavioral sciences, have tried to promote the approach to the patient as a person. Though much praised, the approach has not gained wide success. Engel and his Rochester school have done as much as or more than any one over the past twenty years to reawaken the old concept of the patient as a person, or as Engle prefers to suggest "as a system."[24] He calls this the "*biopsychosocial* medical model," and has termed medical practice based on his model "systems medicine." Such a system-oriented model sees body and mind reciprocally influencing each other, continuously reacting and responding to change. Such a model overcomes the limitations of dualism (which makes the body a puppet hanging from the strings of the mind) and reductionism (which treats body and mind equally as machinery). For Engel it replaces a simple cause-and-effect explanation with "reciprocal causal" models: "The dominant model of disease today is biomedical, with molecular biology its basic scientific discipline. . . . The biomedical model not only requires that disease be dealt with as an entity independent of social behavior, it also demands that behavioral aberrations be explained on the basis of disordered somatic (biochemical or neurophysiological) processes."

As Engel points out, the biomedical model has acquired the status of a dogma. He does not trace the reductionistic biomedical model back very far, but accepts Rasmussen's idea that the notion of a separate soul and body was a concession to the Church and that the resulting dualism left doctor to repair the body and the Church to investigate mind behavior, religion, and the soul.[25]

In accepting a relatively short-lived interpretation of how the biomedical model became established, Engel may stray, but he is an eloquent proponent of how indispensable the psychic and psychosocial extensions are to any definition of disease. Along with Fabrega, Cassell, Lipowski,[26] and others, he has emphasized a wide definition of disease:

> Thus, the biochemical defect may determine certain characteristics of the disease, but not necessarily the point in time when the person falls ill or accepts the sick role or the status of a patient. . . .
>
> The behavior of the physician and the relationship between patient and physician powerfully influence therapeutic outcome for better or for worse.

Engel comments on the importance of understanding the social, personal, and other determinants that make the person seek medical help and accept the status of being a patient. He asks us to probe into

24. Engel, G. L., The need for a new medical model: A challenge for biomedicine, *Science* 196:129–36, 1977.

25. Rasmussen, H., Medical education: Revolution or reaction, *Pharos* 38:53–59, 1975.

26. Fabrega, A behavioral framework; Cassell, E. J., The nature of suffering and the goals of medicine, *NEJM* 306:639–45, 1982; Lipowski, Z. S., Psychosocial aspects of disease, *Ann. Intern. Med.* 71:1197–1206, 1969.

reasons why some people feel pain while others regard similar sensations as everyday events.

Systems medicine redefines health, disease, illness, and disability in terms of the intactness of each component and the ability to function on several hierarchical levels. For Engel a peptic ulcer would not simply be a break in the lining of the stomach, but would be seen as the end result of a breakdown in a system, in a person with a specific social, emotional, and economic status. Thus a change in a person's social environment (getting fired or promoted, for example) "impacts first on psychological functions, e.g. perceptions and appraisal." Engel writes persuasively, but his intellectual arguments sometimes make such hard reading that his approach may not have gained wider acceptance because of the complexity of his concepts.

Hard science versus soft science. It may also be that physicians recognize how little any of us can do about social systems. After all, surveying the social cataclysms of Europe and Asia over the past fifty years, physicians cannot be blamed for feeling that social sciences have made little difference to our world. They cannot be faulted for seeking in their medical practice the reassurances of hard science. When a physician turns to the study of disease, he is delighted at how vastly scientific quantification techniques have improved his knowledge and practice. I know no more today about why an alcoholic wants to drink than I did thirty years ago, but now at least I can plumb his pancreas with a scope to lay out its ducts, and I can outline its contour with computed tomography. Physicians pour over their scientific journals for explanations of disease and how they can treat it, but put aside as too soft material that talks about persons and society. Physicians are pragmatists who want information to help care for their patients. They have little patience—and little time—for matters which help them merely to understand their patients. Engel's systems approach would mean too wholehearted a surrender to a world in which the physician has to consider equally patients and their diseases.

It is extraordinary that physicians in daily practice recognize the importance of these matters, but have not been trained to deal with them. Like lawyers fresh out of law school who have studied the Constitution and legal theory, they are ill equipped to accept the reality of plea bargaining. In his medical career and in his hospital training in acute diseases, the medical student or resident learns little but the care of the acute illness. The person remains a phantom, until people begin to turn up in the office.

Humanity and humanities in medicine. Matters are sometimes made too complex. Common sense is what is needed and possibly only when a good deal of money is funneled into trying to construct a social model of disease will real progress be made. Meanwhile we can wonder that so little happens in the medical schools and so much more happens in daily practice.

Even so, practicing physicians gradually come to understand how important is the patient's experience of his illness, what it means to him, and how he feels about it. Lipowski put it in terms of threat, loss, relief, and insignificance:

> Any attempt to understand why the patient feels and acts in a particular manner must include an inquiry into his subjective interpretation of what is happening to him—and to his personal meaning of events related to his illness. . . . In general, the more the meaning of disease and its symptoms is influenced by unconscious factors, the more irrational, idiosyncratic, and unpredictable is the patient's overt response likely to be.[27]

In other words, if I get sick I worry about the threat to my continued existence and I anticipate bodily harm, worry about whether I will lose part of my body or its function. Obviously I will worry about what is most important to me; an athlete will feel differently about a stiff neck than an intellectual.

That is why novelists and other writers are so important for physicians; they may not help us understand disease any better, but they explain to us what it means to be sick, tell us something about the inner life of the patient and how he communicates to others what he feels. They explore that other world, where the physicist cannot go, where the poet can explain death and daily life better than the scientist. The novelist can help the physician come to terms with many hard problems by giving him distance, allowing the physician to reflect on life and death without having to act on what he thinks.

To read an X-ray, to interpret its lights and shadows, requires training and experience, knowledge of much more than what is seen. To read a poem, as Victor Erlich has emphasized, requires more than seeing the work in front of you.[28] The more poems you have read, the richer your responses, and the more meaning you will derive. To read a poem, he points out, requires as much experience as to read an X-ray, though other doctors might not agree. To understand a patient's history—his story—a physician does not need to have read Henry James or Dostoeyevsky, but the physician who has enlarged his empathy and his understanding of people by his experience in the

27. Lipowski, Psychosocial aspects of disease.

28. Erlich, V., Literature, memory, and medicine. Lecture at Yale Univ. Sch. Med., April 18, 1985.

world of books should be more aware of tones and shades, nuances that a less well-read physician might pass by.

Pain and suffering. Cassell reemphasizes how suffering can come from physical symptoms, from their treatment, and from the knowledge of "an impending destruction of the person."[29] Fitzgerald writes, "Of course all life is a process of breaking down. . . . There is another sort of blow that comes from within—that you don't feel until it's too late to do anything about it, until you realize with finality that in some regard you will never be as good a man again."[30] Cassell is careful to distinguish between pain and the suffering it causes and, like other good clinicians, he knows that pain from a *known* source can be borne with much more equanimity than pain of unknown origin. That is why the studies of pain relief in a laboratory have so little practical meaning to us; a subject bearing the pain produced by an investigator has quite a different sensation from the patient with pain in his belly that he does not understand:

> Patients can writhe in pain from kidney stones and by their own admission not be suffering, because they "know what it is"; they may also report considerable suffering from apparently minor discomfort when they do not know its source. . . .
>
> In summary, people in pain frequently report suffering from the pain when they feel out of control, when the pain is overwhelming, when the source of the pain is unknown, when the meaning of the pain is dire, or when the pain is chronic.

Cassell reemphasizes the importance of the person who feels the pain. For many people suffering comes from injuries to their integrity and from the perception that they will not ever again be what they were. Cassell gives us a clue to how the placebo might work: "Recovery from suffering often involves help, as though people who have lost parts of themselves can be sustained by the personhood of others until their own recovers. This is one of the latent functions of the physicians: to lend strength. A group too may lend strength."

The Metaphors of Disease

Many physicians assume that what is applicable to disease will some day be applicable to illness because of their faith in the scientific method. Because of the triumphs of cell biology and of genetic engineering physicians more than ever apply the wrong analytic tools to the study of illness and even now look for structural changes.

29. Cassell, The nature of suffering.
30. Fitzgerald, F. S., quoted in Lefton, Chronic disease.

The prevailing metaphor of medicine—doctor as scientist or soldier—lead to the metaphor of disease as a physical object, an alien invader. *The Body Snatchers* catches the tone: the aliens convert the human body, outwardly unchanged, to their own uses. People become alien to themselves. The seed pods are the source of disease. The alien invader we can see and measure is all that counts. What the patient tells us, what we hear, is not reliable because he has already been contaminated.

The patient is the witness to some of the events going on in himself, however unknowing a receptacle he often proves. The problem, of course, is that he has to interpret them to a physician immersed in a medical culture. There must be as much emphasis on the ear as on the eye. To attain that equality, however, may prove a very long task because of what Rorty sees as the inherent reliance on seeing in Western culture.[31] The metaphor of the mind's eye, the eye of faith, reminds us that the metaphor of medicine is indeed the eye, the favorite of all the senses. In some ways the eye has become its own icon, worshipped for itself rather than for the person, illness, or suffering it should bring us back to.

Kleinman calls our attention to Wittgenstein's metaphor for scientific language as straight regular streets with uniform houses, which he contrasts with ordinary language as a maze of little streets, of old and new houses: "Our language can be seen as an ancient city: a maze of little streets and squares, of old and new houses, and of houses with additions from various periods; and this surrounded by a multitude of new boroughs with straight regular streets and uniform houses."[32] Kleinman shifts the metaphor to medical theory which pays attention to the "wide, well-designed and clearly mapped suburban avenues" of biophysical science. We pay only "somewhat embarrassed attention" [to] "this archaic route of medicine which strikes us as most like the twisting, narrow, unmapped streets and clutter of old and new houses of the ancient inner city."

Diagnosis: The Eye and the Ear

The patient has to tell his doctor about his illness, but some doctors and some patients find too much conversation too personal. It is curious how intimate conversation or talking seems to be, even to the visually minded generation. In a college seminar titled "Thinking about Medicine" I asked the students to imagine being a patient. The students had no objection to their bodies being probed or even photo-

31. Rorty, R., *Philosophy and the mirror of nature*, Princeton: Princeton University Press, 1979, p. 38.
32. Kleinman, A., Medicine's symbolic reality, *Inquiry* 16:206–13, 1973.

graphed, but the notion that their words would be recorded or taped seemed an intrusion of their privacy. Almost as if the words were a reflection of the mind and they were in their minds, not in their bodies, they objected to having their dialogue with the doctor recorded. "That's too private," one of them complained. "I don't need to let my doctor know what I am thinking." The duality expressed in such observations is clear, but is also paradoxical that physician and patient alike should maintain that reserve of privacy which says that the thoughts as reflected in talk are not important to the understanding of disease. For many people, talk is intimate; the tongue seems to have a direct connection with the thoughts, closer than the spleen. If I tell you what I am thinking or what I fear, you know me, more than if you biopsy my liver, hold my heart in your hands, or read my EEG.

Seeing and talking. Such reserve may be one of the reasons why physicians talk a lot about tumors and what to do about them and so little about patients. Talk is left to the social workers, psychiatrists, and —one hopes—the nursing staff. Yet all one has to do is ask to find that everyone knows the complaint is more than just the disease. Still, in their conferences physicians ignore what they cannot see. At the gastrointestinal conferences at Yale, for example, the pathologist and radiologist are always in attendance to teach us about image and structure; but the social worker is not there, and the psychiatrist is almost never invited. The participants want hard facts and visual images, to learn all they can about technological matters to apply to their patients. They "know" the rest and do not need to discuss it. The message to those in training is "Get the image." Yet few older clinicians can agree with the idea that all diseases will be explainable on the basis of a switch which is turned on or off by some gene.

Imaging techniques and concepts of disease. There is much to the lure of technology for physicians, particularly when it gives them little printouts or pictures to show each other. Those little icons of disease, the X-rays and echoes and scans, give an image to the pains of the patient, but one which has been sterilized and flattened. The image carries with it none of the sorrow or apprehension that sounds so anguishing when the live person talks of his pain. It is much easier to focus on a film in an office far from the patient than to listen to the patient. When the patient is through talking, we have only the memory of what he said. When he has been to the X-ray (now imaging) department, we have a permanent record and a picture.

Physicians need to examine how their concepts of disease change when we come to depend upon such imaging techniques to show us the disease rather than simply inferring the diagnosis from hearing the patient's complaints. It is the switch from the ear to the eye. Complaints are evanescent, at least to the physician; they are words uttered, listened to, which quickly "float away on the air," in Walter Ong's lovely phrase. An image, whether X-ray, echo, or endoscopic photograph, or even a number from a laboratory test, is far more permanent. The image or the number fixes the disease, to give it a reality which makes physicians think of it as a thing.

To be sure physicians have always delighted in giving names to complaints, even in ancient times. In the *Republic* III Plato comments:

> Just because, by indolence and a habit of life such as we have been describing, men fill themselves with waters and winds, as if their bodies were a marsh, compelling the ingenious sons of Asclepius to find more names for diseases, such as flatulence and catarrh; is not this, too, a disgrace?
>
> "Yes," he said, "they do certainly give very strange and new fangled names to diseases."

To many physicians the ulcer displayed on a film becomes much more important, something to act on with more assurance, more than when they deduce it from the patient's story. Yet if I listen to a patient with a good story for a duodenal ulcer, I can treat him "symptomatically" and he will probably get better. There are even advantages in that approach for him: if I have not "proven" the diagnosis by recording it on endoscopic or X-ray film, his life insurance company will regard the diagnosis as unproven and so nonexistent. Once portrayed on X-ray or endoscopy, the ulcer may cost my patient 5 percent more of his life insurance payments, at least for a while. The insurance company also relies on the eye more than the ear. Everyone wants to prove by seeing. Indeed one of the dangers of paying for diagnoses in the so-called diagnostic-related groups may turn out to be that physicians will do more procedures rather than fewer, to "confirm" by images what the ear has already heard. Physicians may even "shoot" for the best-paying diagnosis.

Over the years I have suggested to physicians that they treat even new-onset ulcer dyspepsia with an anti-ulcer program for ten days, postponing diagnostic tests for a while and investigating only those whose pain has not relented. Academicians complain in rejoinder that medicine is a science—or should be—"We must know what we are treating." They feel uncomfortable not "proving" what is present by seeing it. Clinicians in practice retort that they will be sued for malpractice if they delay the diagnosis for even ten days, although such a delay may be meaningless for the outlook in cancer.

Seeing the "disease" makes physicians think about it quite differently than when we talk about it. Different imaging techniques may even give us a different concept of a disease. To me duodenal ulcer by X-ray is somehow abstract, a black and white shadow with no close re-lation to real life. By endoscopy, face to face so to speak, a duodenal ulcer looks just like any other sore.

The imaging explosion is displaying disease in an ever-expanding way. But when physicians begin to think of a disease only in terms of its anatomical expression, only when it is "proven," they run the risk of thinking of a disease only as a thing. They run the risk of ignoring complaints, pain, or suffering, at least until they can see them on a screen. That notion is reinforced by their colleagues, who also accept a diagnosis only when they can see it. Gradually more and more dis-eases take on the aspects of an object, in philosophical terms are reified. The primacy of anatomy is once again being asserted, in a way not dissimilar from that when anatomists were first dissecting out and naming what they found at the examination of cadavers.

Cholecystitis. The need to see the disease has affected the diagnostic process in acute cholecystitis.[33] The old-fashioned clinician, who felt that he could recognize acute cholecystitis by its characteristic history and positive physical findings, is now surprised to read of the unreli-ability of clinical findings when they are compared to ultrasound and radionuclide study. A high percentage of patients who are considered to have acute cholecystitis on a clinical basis prove not to have it when imaging techniques are applied. Such disparity between the clinical diagnosis and the imaging procedure may be real—and it may turn out that physicians should make diagnoses only by images. On the other hand such an approach may simply reflect the ignorance or in-experience of a clinician or, just as plausibly, his abdication before the diagnostic images. If students and residents are taught to recognize acute cholecystitis only by positive images, that will greatly influence the way in which the disorder is conceived and detected. That is, if the resident is convinced that the only way to make the diagnosis of acute cholecystitis is by radionuclide scan, that is what he will do in the emergency room and later in practice. He will give up trying to make the diagnosis clinically and order the scan instead. Presumably a wider and wider range of poorly characterized abdominal complaints will be subjected to IDA scanning as the best way to make the diagno-sis. That indeed may be correct, but at present the skeptic will wonder whether the clinical diagnosis (nondiagnosis really) was carefully thought about before the test was ordered. If anyone with pain from

33. Spiro, H. M., Burrell, M. I., and Zeman, R. K., Clinical-radiologic perspectives on gallbladder and bileduct imaging, in *Radiology of the gallbladder and bile ducts*, ed. R. Berk, J. Ferrucci, and G. Leopold, Philadelphia: Saunders, 1983.

knee to chest undergoes an IDA scan to rule out acute cholecystitis, then the clinical "diagnosis" is being improperly compared to the imaging technique. In this way the concept of acute cholecystitis as a clinically detectable disease grows even weaker. Worse, the idea that a clinician can learn anything useful from talking to the patient appears ever more ludicrous.

Classifications and models tell us something about the concerns of a society or culture. For example, in a wet country rain is particularized as shower, mist, downpour, sprinkle, and in many other terms that would be meaningless to desert nomads. Ozick describes the scorn of the Eastern European Jew for the Christian categorization of knives: "By them they got sword, they got lance, they got halberd . . . cutlass, pike, rapier, foil, ten dozen more."[34]

In talking about our diagnostic errors, western physicians have room for only Type I and Type II categories, based on the presence or absence of detectable disease. There is, for example, no Type III, which might be finding on an imaging technique a "disease" that doesn't really matter to the patient, such as a hemangioma of the liver; or Type IV, over-emphasizing the importance of an asymptomatic finding such as primary biliary cirrhosis about which so little, except for liver transplant, can be done. Such emphasis only on visible abnormalities, with no concern for their significance, tells us a great deal about the nature of doctors' concerns.

Observer variation. Observer variation is not something that we need consider in great detail, but it sets an important limit to medical vision. The term refers to the disagreement that arises when different observers look at the same object, and try to describe what they have seen. If, for example, three physicians look through an endoscope at an "ulcer," they will disagree roughly a third of the time about what they see, or at least will describe it in very different terms. Ten pathologists getting together to decide what they saw on a series of slides disagreed among themselves 20 to 30 percent of the time.[35] Although I have not seen such a study, I suspect that the smaller the object studied, or the more powerful and complex the apparatus placed between the observer and the observed, the less likely there is to be observer variation, if only because there are fewer points to describe. Presumably few would disagree about a circle, for example.

In any event, identifying the reasons for error in seeing and de-

34. Ozick, C., Puttermessen, in *Levitation*, New York: Dutton, p. 34.
35. Riddell, R. H., Goldman, H., Ransohoff, D. F., et al., Dysplasia in inflammatory bowel disease, *Human Path.* 14:931–68, 1983.

scribing something has become a science of its own. Rose and Barker describe four components:[36] (1) within-observer variation, referring to the individual's inconsistency in reporting the same observation; (2) between-observer variation, a systematic component of error due to individual differences in criteria and we may add, visual powers; (3) random variation in what is being observed at different times (blood pressure measurements will vary around the subject's mean blood pressure from time to time); and finally (4) biased variation in the observed because of many outside factors. But what these comments tell us is that even when a sense as transparently accurate as the eye is used, there is still always observer variation. Observer variation not only enters into seeing, but enters just as much into telling or describing what has been seen.

Fixing the idea of a disease. Images freeze the idea of disease. Looking at the "disease" on the scan or film is quicker and easier than getting an idea of it from the story that the patient tells. Any new understanding must come from improvement in techniques rather than from reflection, conversation, or analysis of the patients themselves. In a way, it is the same shift that occurs when language changes from a purely oral communication to a written script, the change from intuition and magic to science and reason.[37] Such a change in medicine has proven extremely valuable, but at the loss of conversation and communication between patient and physician. As Ong has pointed out, speaking is the consciousness of another person.[38] Sound penetrates the ear. Because the sound is so quickly gone, we have to pay attention to it as it occurs. Sight, on the other hand, and its frozen counterpart, the image, is more permanent. We can look at the image again and again. It is easier to bring the picture back to the mind's eye than to the ear. To be sure we could tape record an interview with the patient, to capture his sound as data, to make the complaint more permanent. Curiously, however, we don't, or at least very few physicians do, except to have a record of informed consent. Even audiotapes have yielded to videotapes. Few physicians, however, have ever thought the patient's words important enough to capture the sound, the complaints of a disease, on tape. It would surely be as easy to tape a patient's recounting of his pains or problems as to reconstruct his image on computed tomographic (CT) scan. But in a sense, as my college students reminded me, it would be a violation of his "privacy" in

36. Rose, G., and Barber, D. S., Observer variation. *Brit. Med. J.* 2:1006–07, 1978.
37. McLuhan, M., *Understanding media*, New York: McGraw Hill, 1964.
38. Ong. W. J., *Interfaces of the word*, Ithaca: Cornell University Press, 1977, p. 125.

a way that looking at his liver is not. We get at the real person when we listen to him. But that takes time.

Listening to the patient brings immediacy, face-to-face contact. There may be a loss of precision, the accuracy of the eye, but so much more is enhanced. Over the telephone? On audiotape? I do not know, but I suspect that the voice is a different one. I listen to the phone quite differently from the way I listen to a person. I must concentrate more. If the physician recognizes that the way in which we ask questions is as important as what the patient will tell us and what we hear, the act of communication will be enhanced. Every patient tells his own story, the story changes a little each time it is told, and it may be told differently to different doctors. For some physicians such variations make the story soft data, not as reliable as the hard copy of the image.

Look at the clinical situation. Where once the patient called the physician to his home, now the patient goes to the physician in hospital or office, each the physician's territory. If he has not already had his secretary give the patient a checklist of symptoms or installed a monitor for a computerized history, the physician has a list of questions at the ready. He knows what he wants to find out, has questioned many patients before, but for the patient the process is, we may assume, a new one. In pain, ill at ease, he is looking for help. Havens emphasizes that even in psychoanalysis, silence can be misinterpreted:

> The physician interrogates the patient, who must be able to understand the questions, ask them of himself, and then report back accurately the answers. . . .
>
> Medical examining, with its heavy emphasis on questions, makes the sharpest subject-object differentiation; we can speak of a maximal psychological distance. Typically, *I* question *you*. The grammatical form is the second person singular, "Are you . . ." or "You are . . .", either questions or descriptions. . . .
>
> If the language that occurs to us is in part a function of our distance from the patient, then we can change our language by changing our distance, just as we can change our distance by changing our language (active empathy).[39]

Images sterilize disease. Modern diagnostic images give the objectivity that current physicians so prize in their model of science, but these images denature and dehumanize disease. Disease becomes abstract. Not only have we lost the complaint of the sick person, but there is no longer any background; no sense beyond sight is required—no smell or touch or hearing. Poetry is emotion "recollected in tranquillity,"

39. Havens, L. L., Explorations in the uses of language in psychotherapy: Simple empathic statements, *Psychiatry* 41:336–44, 1978.

Wordsworth said. Disease is as trapped on film as emotions are trapped in poetry, and it is made more endurable for the physician. Once the radiologist had to touch the patient to X-ray him, but now the techniques of computed tomography and magnetic resonance imaging make it possible for images of the patient's whole body to be reconstructed in an "imaging department," without the radiologist ever seeing the patient. Indeed, given the precision of these instruments the imaging physician could be a thousand miles away as long as the image can be transmitted over the wires. The physician turns to the radiologist for his answer, often more as a supplicant than a colleague. No one puts the whole patient back together after his complaints have been put on the screen, fractured into an MRI, US, CT, IDA, and all the rest of the alphabetical tests.

Diseases have become linear, studied by one test after another, in a sense sequestered, and few of us can put the whole picture back together again. That is surely one reason why "holistic" practitioners are becoming so popular.

A very important function of the physician in the age of imaging will be to act as the interpreter of the patient's complaints, as the mediator between man and machines, between complaints and images. This should prove even more important with improved technology. First, of course, the physician has to hear what the patient has to say. There are blind physicians, but are there any deaf ones? Presumably a deaf person could become a fine radiologist or even a surgeon, but he cannot break through that communication barrier that we instinctively feel when someone cannot hear what we want to tell him. Try reading poetry to someone hard-of-hearing. The voice tells so much. Physicians are hypnotized by images. Physicians should look on images as freeing them from the constraints of the physical examination, giving more time to listen, to talk with the person, but they don't. They see more patients or order more studies.

The live theater is a different experience from the movies just as the live patient is different from his image. Marshall McLuhan put it vividly: "Suppose that, instead of displaying the Stars and Stripes, we were to write the words 'American flag' across a piece of cloth and to display that. While the symbols would convey the same meaning, the effect would be quite different."[40]

Grand Rounds as a reflection. "Grand Rounds" gives some clues to the changes in medicine. They began, as the name implies, literally as a tour around the wards by the chief physician and his associates. The patient was the center of the discussion, even if he might be ignored

40. McLuhan, *Understanding media.*

once his problem had been resolved, serving only as a focus for discussion. Then, becoming unwieldy as a teaching exercise because too many physicians came to such rounds, Grand Rounds were moved to an amphitheatre. At first patients were brought to the conference, so that physicians could still have someone to talk to, to listen to, to see. The discussion was personal, oral, informed, and patient-centered.

Gradually the aim of the conference shifted from a *problem* patient whose disease might be explored and subsequent therapy improved by discussion, to an *interesting* patient whose disease was used to focus discussion intended to improve the knowledge and skills of physicians. At that point the particular patient ceased to be of any importance, and his disease took precedence. It was the shift from a patient to a case. At the same time concern for the patient's rights and privacy made displaying him at a conference seem a breach of that privacy. Less and less time was allowed for talking to the patient, until he became an icon of himself, a case, present like the American flag to show that there was a patient/person somewhere in the background. Anyone could have been put into a bed to represent the patient, for all of the good it did to bring the patient to Grand Rounds. That is probably why the patient is no longer present—no one knows what to do with him!

From the case it is not far to statistics, organs, and the apparatus of reductionism. Today, Grand Rounds in most hospitals have become lectures, written presentations which are read aloud. Often enough there is no longer even the pretense of a patient presentation. The speaker stands and talks, pointing to his slides projected on a screen and too often reading his slides as much as any paper in front of him: "Don't worry if you can't read the slides. They're to remind me what to say. They're not for you at all!" The audience is being read to, not talked to. Yet the logic of a written paper is quite different from the construction of a talk to an audience that is supposed to be listening as much as reading. Grand Rounds now usually partake of the written tradition, not the oral one. After many rounds written summaries—handouts—are distributed for later review.

The physician relies on the written word almost as much as on the image. "Give me the reference!" has become the watchword. Physicians have only to see something in print to believe it, while hearing it means a lot less. I suppose that is not so very different from other people. My wife and I were on an island not too long ago, walking to breakfast along a village road. Behind us we heard the hum of a car coming along slowly. Neither of us turned, but then we heard the car veer off along a road to the left. She looked back to confirm with her eyes what our ears had told us. "I wanted to be sure," she explained.

The religion of vision. Meyer emphasizes the American "religion of vision": "The English ear has been killed by the American eye, the divine work has been usurped by the divine vision."[41] The eagle with its eagle eye, the mystic eye of our seal emblazoned on the dollar bill, the Statue of Liberty with its lamp, all these, Meyer emphasizes, tell us how everything in America relies on, lives by, the eye. From the early poets whose religious experiences occurred in visual settings to Emerson, who called the American a "transparent eyeball," the same theme runs to the present-day emphasis on television. Meyer points out the American passion for vision. The concept of the word, the mysteries of the unseen, have been bleached out by the light of the television set.

But the reliance on vision is not strictly American. The entire scientific approach depends on what Ong has called "hypervisualism," the notion that all the sensations can be reduced to vision through devices such as charts or measurements.[42] The image isolates the patient from the physician, just as sight isolates and freezes, but sound penetrates and, as Ong puts it, "pours" into the listener. Scientific medicine isolates the patient from the physician, lets the physician—ever more the technologist or test-orderer—be silent, like the proverbial kind old surgeon. What physician has not felt a great triumph at seeing on X-ray film what he had predicted would be there? The detective story is solved, the problem literally visualized. But listening to the same unraveling of the story, learning from the patient the cause of his pain does not give most physicians the same thrill. The Greeks said that the eye was for accuracy but the ear was for truth. Vision demands preconception and organization, but sound demands an even more harmonious putting together of what the patient is telling us.

The physician looks for disease rather than listens to the patient. Yet illness, the patient's complaint, can only be understood by listening to what he says. It is detected by the ear. Disease, what the physician can find, is proven by the image produced for the eye. The diagnosis of illness comes from listening, but the detection of disease from the image. The words of the physician, or even the symbols of his words and presence may, we shall find, be helpful in the treatment of illness, but technology and drugs are crucial to recognition and treatment of disease. Illness, then, is tied up with complaints and with what the patient says, what the doctor hears rather than what he sees. No one can "see" an illness. The visual metaphors which equate

41. Meyer, W. E., The American religion of vision, *Christian Century*, 16 Nov. 1983: 1045–47.
42. Ong, *Interfaces of the word.*

"knowing" with "seeing" are universal in medicine. In writing of "The Chemistry of the Mind" Wagner remarked, not recognizing the paradox, "We now have a new set of eyes that permit us to begin to examine the chemistry of the mind."

Modern physicians do not listen to the difference between "I *see* what you say," and "I *hear* what you say," as Ong has suggested. Indeed students learn about diseases, by reading references and textbooks, but they learn about caring by watching caring physicians in something between an apprenticeship where they do, and a discipleship, again to use Ong's terms, where they learn to say. Physicians have to recognize that images can free them from the constraints of the physical examination, thus giving them more time to listen to the patient. Listening is much harder work than seeing; it takes time, concentration, and active participation. But physicians need to listen as much as to look, to make all senses work together.

6

Reported Responses
to Placebo:
The Placebo Effect

T
he placebo response and the placebo effect make

up the fourth act of the drama, but the two scenes are separate. The effect, upon disease, is different from the response, what the patient feels. The placebo effect is the climax of the drama. One of the first to work in this field, Wolf, defined the placebo effect as "any effect attributable to a pill, potion, or procedure, but not to its pharmacodynamic or specific properties."[1] Such a definition falls short owing to the fact that we can never be sure that all the "effects" or "properties" can be measured. Brody defines the placebo effect as "the change in the patient's condition that is attributable to the symbolic import of the healing intervention rather than to the intervention's specific pharmacologic or physiologic effects."[2] In chapter 2, following Grunbaum, I discussed the problems inherent in using the words *specific* or *nonspecific*, which I call attention to here. Fisher distinguishes the placebo *response*, which is the behavioral change in the subject receiving the pill, from the placebo *effect*, that part of the change which can be attributed to the *symbolic* effect of being given a medication.[3] As the placebo affects the patient, and not the disease, it is very important to distinguish response from effect. When Brody uses the term "patient's condition", I suspect that he means disease and not a more existential state. I would prefer the "patient's complaints."

1. Wolf, S., The pharmacology of placebos, *Pharmacologic Rev.* 11:689–704, 1959.
2. Brody, H., The lie that heals: The ethics of giving placebos, *Ann. Intern. Med.* 97:112–18, 1982.
3. Fisher, S., The placebo reactor: Thesis, antithesis, synthesis, and hypothesis, *Dis. Nerv. Syst.* 28:510–15, 1967.

There are then two parts to the placebo effect. The first and most dramatic is the placebo response, which is attributed to suggestibility or what the act of receiving a placebo does to the illness component of the disease. The second has to do with remission of disease. As I have earlier emphasized, most diseases get better on their own and if the patient gets a pill or potion at the time he feels the worst, then the placebo or other pill may receive credit for natural improvement. Some diseases, even cancer, undergo spontaneous remission, and we must always require more than a single anecdote to assure us that a response is predictable, not just a rare coincidence. With the distinction between response and effect in mind, let me review some of the published claims for what the placebo can do.

Preexisting Symptoms

In the early 1960s, when ideas about informed consent had not yet precluded certain kinds of psychological experiments, Green noted that the side effects of placebos in controlled trials were almost "invariably similar in type to the side-effects of the active drug itself."[4] He thought that those side effects might have depended on what the investigator was looking for, but he also wondered whether preexisting complaints which might otherwise have gone unnoted were being regarded as side effects. He and his colleagues then told a very large number of people that they were trying to determine the side effects of a new drug, but did not tell those subjects that they were getting placebos nor of the expected side effects. As any gastroenterologist might have suspected, gastrointestinal complaints loomed large beforehand: heartburn, nausea, and abdominal pain were not infrequent; dizziness, blurred vision, dry mouth, palpitation, urinary frequency, and drowsiness were also reported. After the subjects had taken the placebo, symptoms that had been present beforehand were much increased in frequency and severity. "The only new symptom elicited by placebos was vomiting." Gastrointestinal complaints became more prominent, along with drowsiness and dizziness, and the complaints increased with the number of placebo pills. Patients in an old-age home grew particularly alarmed about their symptoms; their nurses suggested that the drugs be stopped because of their "toxic" effects. In this very illuminating paper Green concluded:

> The ability of placebos to intensify the apparent severity of such pre-treatment symptoms and to elicit them in others in whom they had not pre-existed, suggest that the active administrating of medication may so focus the subject's attention introspectively that some

4. Green, D. M., Pre-existing conditions, placebo reactions, and "side effects," *Ann. Intern. Med.* 60:255–65, 1964.

complaints previously given little or no attention are magnified to a degree where they become regarded as "side effects" of the medication being given.[5]

The placebo response in clinical trials is influenced by the severity of the initial complaint and by associated complaints.[6]

Cancer

One of the most dramatic cases referred to by several authors, at least in reference and footnote, turns out to be less impressive on review. The author was a psychologist, Bruno Klopfer, who told the story in his 1957 presidential address to the Society for Projective Techniques.[7] Klopfer was not the physician caring for the patient, but quoted the account by a Dr. Philip West, who is otherwise unidentified. A patient of unknown age, "Mr. Wright had a generalized far-advanced malignancy involving the lymph nodes, lymphosarcoma. . . . Huge tumor masses, the size of oranges, were in the neck, axillas, groins, chest and abdomen."

The patient was given a course of Krebiozen, a "cancer cure" of the 1950s, with great enthusiasm and, after one injection, the physician writes, "What a surprise was in store for me! I had left him febrile, gasping for air, completely bedridden. Now, here he was, walking around the ward chatting happily with the nurses. . . . The tumor masses had melted like snowballs on a hot stove and in only these few days, they were half their original size!" Reports, however, began to appear that Krebiozen was of no value:

> This disturbed our Mr. Wright considerably as the weeks wore on. Although he had no special training, he was, at times, reasonably logical and scientific in his thinking. He began to lose faith in his last hope which so far had been life-saving and left nothing to be desired. As the reported results became increasingly dismal, his faith waned and after two months of practically perfect health, he relapsed to his original state, and became very gloomy and miserable.

At this point the physician

> decided to take the chance and play the quack. So deliberately lying, I told him not to believe what he read in the papers, the drug was really most promising after all. . . .

5. Ibid.
6. Schachtel, B. P., Fillingim, J. M., Beiter, D. J., et al., Rating scales for analgesics in sore throat, *Clin. Pharm. Therapeutics* 36:151–56, 1984.
7. Klopfer, B., Psychological variables in human cancer, *J. Projective Techniques* 21:331–40, 1957.

I administered the first injection of the doubly potent, fresh preparation—consisting of fresh water and nothing more. The results of this experiment were quite unbelievable to us at the time. . . . Tumor masses melted, chest fluid vanished, he became ambulatory.

The water injections were continued, since they worked such wonders, the patient remaining symptom-free over two months. Then, "the final AMA announcement appeared in the press—Nationwide tests show Krebiozen to be a worthless drug in the treatment of cancer. . . . Within a few days of this report, Mr. Wright was readmitted to the hospital in extremis . . . and he succumbed in less than two days."

Obviously there is no objective data to rely on in such a report, beyond the second-hand testimonial. Not only is the physician unknown, we have no evidence beyond the recounting of the experience, and it is easy to conjecture that much of the report was enthusiastic interpretation. To be sure the patient felt better, but it cannot be helpful to carry on, without better documentation, the notion that placebos can dissolve the objective manifestations of cancer, any more than to accept other preposterous claims made on behalf of other therapies.

In the general cheer of the *New Haven Register* of December 25, 1984, a report appeared of a woman who had lived much longer than had been expected after the diagnosis of a pancreatic cancer. She was alive after two years, and as most patients die within six months, I read on. It turned out that the diagnosis was not made by biopsies, but by palpation, a technique which is no more accurate than tossing a coin. The patient was grateful, but I must remain skeptical.

Spontaneous remission. Sometimes, for ill-understood and unpredictable reasons, the growth of some cancers slows and a very few even disappear. Those occurrences are so rare as to defy classification, but that rarity raises doubt about most reported "cures" of cancer. In a remarkable review, *Spontaneous Regression of Cancer,* Drs. Everson and Cole of the University of Illinois College of Medicine in 1966 brought together 176 reports of cancers which had disappeared or at least grown smaller for some time.[8] They recorded only cases of cancer which had undergone adequate histologic documentation of malignancy. They defined spontaneous regression as "partial or complete disappearance of malignant tumor in the absence of all treatment" or in the presence of inadequate treatment. More than half the collected remissions occurred in cancers of the kidney, the nervous

8. Everson, T. C., and Cole, W. H., Spontaneous regression of cancer, Philadelphia: Saunders, 1966, p. 4.

system, skin (malignant melanoma), and the uterus and ovaries (choriocarcinoma). Unfortunately it was impossible even for those assiduous physicians to determine how long the spontaneous regression lasted or whether it was permanent; reports usually were published shortly after the improvement had been noted, a testimony to the enthusiasm even of doctors for the miraculous. The reasons for the spontaneous regressions were, of course, uncertain; Everson and Cole considered hormonal influences most likely.

Such an important reminder that spontaneous regression does occur suggests the need for much caution in accepting the efficacy of any therapeutic measure which purports to cure cancer, orthodox or alternative: "The occurrence of spontaneous regression of cancer demonstrates the need for caution in the assessment of the value of chemotherapeutic and unorthodox therapeutic measures in isolated 'cures' of cancer."

They quote Dunphy, who stated: "It is obvious that occasional temporary regressions or arrests of tumors cannot be interpreted as evidence of a successful response to a particular agent unless it is consistently observed in many different cases."[9] That consistency is what is lacking in most claims of miraculous cures whether by faith healing or alternative forms of therapy. Some cancers do get smaller, some do stand still, and it is consistency that we must require from the proponents of any specific cure.

While thinking about such matters, I had occasion to see a middle-aged woman, a former alcoholic, who had undergone abdominal exploration in another city for a mass in her pancreas which had been thought to be a cancer. As biopsies of the mass at operation failed to reveal any malignancy, the pancreas was not removed. Two pathologists at separate university hospitals reviewing the biopsies agreed that no cancer was present. Returning to Connecticut, the patient came for another opinion. She was healthy, worked in her garden every day, and had abstained from alcohol for the past several months. She had even gained some weight, a highly unlikely probability for someone with pancreatic cancer. Another computed tomographic scan of her pancreas showed that the tumor in the pancreas, whether benign or malignant, had grown somewhat larger. Two pathologists at Yale then reviewed the biopsy specimens and both agreed that cancer was present, to the consternation of the patient and those taking care of her. The biopsy specimen was then sent on to pathologists at another hospital specializing in cancer, but they did not agree with the diagnosis.

9. Dunphy, J. E., Some observations on the natural behaviour of cancer in men, *NEJM* 242:167–72, 1950.

In the meantime she agreed with her physicians that the circumstances warranted no radical form of therapy because the outlook for pancreatic cancer was so bad, the diagnosis still so uncertain, and the fruits of chemotherapy even more so. Still she elected to go to California to what she called a "fruit and nut" establishment. There she underwent a course of quasi-holistic therapy. Returning to Connecticut, she underwent another computed tomographic scan two months after the first, and the mass was considerably smaller. She has continued to do well.

Certainly this case exemplifies the uncertainties of medicine, but all of us treating her have many questions. Is the response, if that is what it must be called, a success of the holistic approach? Does it represent simply misdiagnosis of cancer? Who knows? But such cases make it very difficult for me to accept the cures claimed by holistic and other practitioners. If that patient lives, as I hope she will, she will no doubt be claimed as a legitimate cure by the California doctors who, after all, told her from the beginning that they accept any diagnosis of cancer made at Yale.

Laboratory Studies

Most writers on the topic accept the idea that placebos can produce impressive physiologic changes, from reduction in blood pressure to a fall in blood sugar levels. The nature of the evidence and the time-frame of many of these observations put them in doubt. Many old reports of placebo response in the laboratory can be regarded with some skepticism. For example, Jospe accepts the notion "that placebos may induce subtle physiological changes that parallel the subjective experiences described by the subject"[10] in the famous study of Wolf and Wolff.[11] Jospe accepts the idea that abdominal discomfort and reddening of the folds of the stomach occurred after "three large imposing-looking red capsules." Review of the original material shows how little can be interpreted, at least in the 1980s. The subject was under considerable stress:

> His behavior during the tests was alert and tense, and following ingestion of certain of the substances which seemed to induce special anxiety, he often noted abdominal cramps and diarrhoea which could not be attributed to the effect of the drug. This disturbance began following an experiment in which he ingested 0.015 gm prostigmine. The cramps and diarrhea in this instance were doubtless due to the pharmacological action of the drug.

10. Jospe, M., *The placebo effect*, Lexington, MA: D. C. Heath, 1978.
11. Wolf, S., and Wolff, H., *Human gastric function*. London: Oxford University Press, 1947.

In order to test whether the prostigmine had a conditioning effect, the investigators decided to give Tom the aforementioned red capsules, which, however, contained "only starch and lactose." Tom's stoma began to blush, "He then noted mild abdominal cramps and an urgent need to defecate. . . . He promptly had one loose stool and his face continued to be red for half an hour. He expressed extreme anxiety regarding the content of the capsules and at this time he was reassured that they contained only milk sugar."

From a vantage point forty years later, we know that lactose produces diarrhea in a large proportion of subjects, and for that reason I find it impossible to conclude that the "placebo" was inactive. This is not to denigrate those studies, but to emphasize the problems associated with evaluating placebo studies either in a laboratory or elsewhere.

In its time the Wolf and Wolff study was important. A modern critical observer might note that changes in the color of the gastric mucosa were made by visual estimate without any concern for observer variation, or without blinding of the observer, so near as can be told. He might conclude that such studies could reflect the intuition or the expectations of the observer as much as changes in the stomach mucosa. He might even note that as Tom was working as a laboratory assistant in the very place where he was being studied, he could not have remained innocent of expectations.

Jospe also accepts the notion that sterile water increased gastric secretion. In fact what Wolf and Wolff found was that the hypodermic injection of 1 cc of sterile water provoked resentment, as the subject "disliked intensely being pricked by hypodermic needles (p. 69)." It was the resentment, and the anger, according to them which produced an increase in gastric secretion of from two to five milliliters. The study was quite important in pointing to the effect of many different agents and emotions on a single stomach. Still, from the standpoint of the 1980s, we cannot accept that injections of water which the subject hated have useful things to show about the placebo. I think that the Wolf and Wolff studies were intended to show the effect of psychic stimuli, not the specific effect of therapeutic stimuli like the placebo, and they should not be overextended.

Subject or patient. There is a world of difference, after all, between a normal subject, who is paid for his time in a laboratory getting pills and reporting his responses, some pleasant and some unpleasant, and the sick patient who comes to a physician for help and who is given a pill to relieve symptoms. There is surely a different context for the subject being given a pill which he is told may make him sleepy or nauseated or give him a headache, and the patient receiving a pill for relief of a symptom. There is much confusion in the literature about these different aspects of the placebo, all "nonphysiological" effects being labeled placebo effects. Indeed a drug which causes unpleasant side effects has sometimes been called a "nocecibo." We must be very careful about accepting such reports, since at least one study has shown that many of the symptoms commonly considered adverse effects of a placebo were present before and were simply magnified by attention to them during study.[12] Placebo responses in the patient with symptoms are really quite a different matter from the responses to a placebo of a subject in a laboratory setting. Almost all patients will prove placebo reactors, if we accept as a placebo effect responding to the physician who is helpful in a positive manner. The psychosocial aspects of illness are manifested in all of us.

Indeed the problem in studying any kind of injection as a placebo has to do with the enormous variability in subjects and patients in the number of injections that they have received before. The chronic pain patient accustomed to receiving injections might react quite differently from someone who has never had many needles before. It is difficult to separate the reaction to the needle from the response to the drug. I am inclined to accept Jospe's comments: "Since the nature of the placebo itself (whether pill or capsule or blue or green or yellow or pink or fluid or injection) does not appear to be the prime determinant of the placebo effect, we must expand our search into other aspects of situations in which placebos are administered."[13]

Effects on Blood Sugar

In *Placebos and the Philosophy of Medicine,*[14] Brody states that "placebos can lower blood sugar levels in diabetics." He refers to a 1967 paper by Singer and Hurwitz,[15] but review of that paper does not permit the implication that a placebo can lower the blood sugar level. The two doctors treated a group of diabetic patients for six months with an active antidiabetic drug, then they gave them a placebo for six months, and finally another trial of active drug was conducted. The exact nature of the succeeding experiments need not concern us. It is of parenthetical interest to note, however, that even in the Boston of the 1960s no attempt at informed consent was thought necessary: "After a six month trial, an identical placebo was substituted without acknowledgement to the patient."

12. Schachtel, Fillingim, Beiter, et al., Rating scales for analgesics.

13. Jospe, *The placebo effect.*

14. Brody, H., *Placebos and the philosophy of medicine*, Chicago: University of Chicago Press, 1980, p. 11.

15. Singer, D. L., and Hurwitz, D., Long-term experience with sulfonylureas and placebo, *NEJM* 277:450–56, 1967.

The point of the paper was that many of the patients maintained very good long-term control of their diabetes on the placebo. The authors were careful to point out, however, that because the patients were in the study, they came regularly to the clinic and had more intense care and a closer relationship with their attending physician. I interpret their observations to show that good care can do as much for some diabetics as some drugs. Such a phenomenon is well known; many insulin-dependent diabetics do well when they lose weight and modify their habits. But nowhere is there the observation that giving a placebo is followed by a lowered blood sugar level, certainly the implication of the statement in Brody's book. That is not to say that a placebo might not lower blood sugar acutely, but that the data to show this was not given in the Singer and Hurwitz study.

What I emphasize by reviewing these papers is that any attempt in the 1980s to evaluate the contribution of placebo therapy should be as rigorous as any other scientific investigation. We should not allow ourselves to state any more or less than any other scientific observer would do. Every physician knows that pain, whether of angina pectoris or duodenal ulcer, will be relieved by placebo or by a caring relationship. Controlled trials emphasize the astonishingly high rate of relief of pain or healing of duodenal ulcer once it comes under observation. We must distinguish the benefit of the care and the concern that the patient gets as inadvertent placebo therapy in controlled clinical trials, such as that of the Boston diabetics, from more objective evidence of physiological effects. We must distinguish, at least for now, the relief that comes from a relationship with a caring person, medical or other, and the specific events evoked by a pill.

Other Disorders

In 1959 Stewart Wolf reviewed a number of reports which at that time convincingly showed that placebos could arrest some disease processes largely through psychosomatic connections,[16] but it is hard to distinguish the importance of suggestion in his reports from the effect of the pills given. He ascribed much of the power of the placebo to the meaningful situation, the circumstances in which the placebo was then, but the data he drew upon would not withstand modern scrutiny.

Some of the "evidence" carried from one paper to another is reminiscent of the lists in *Genesis*. A lot of names are listed, but they don't mean a great deal. For example, Brody quotes Bourne: "The follow-

16. Wolf, S., The pharmacology of placebos, *Pharmacologic Review* 11:689–704, 1959.

ing list of conditions in which placebos have been shown to produce relief: cough, mood changes, angina pectoris, headache, seasickness, anxiety, hypertension, status asthmaticus, depression, and the common cold."[17] Bourne's 1971 paper, in fact, simply quotes a very famous paper by Beecher in 1955![18] Beecher's paper gives traceable references for pain, cough, mood changes, angina pectoris, and the common cold; there are no traceable references for headache or seasickness. Bourne simply adds status asthmaticus, hypertension, depression, and hyperglycemia without citing evidence. Bourne, however, makes the following very important point about all diseases in which placebo is said to help: "In these diseases the percentage of patients receiving relief is not so high, but in virtually every study a considerable number of patients are helped by placebo medication. A study that shows no response to placebo might almost be suspected of lack of objectivity on that ground alone."

Overinterpretation. An example of overstatement by implication occurs in Sissela Bok's book *Lying*, in which she states: "Worst of all, those children who cannot tolerate antibiotics may have severe reactions, sometimes fatal, to such unnecessary medication."[19] That is certainly true of antibiotics, as the reference she quotes states, whether used as placebo or not.[20] Certainly antibiotics should not be used as a placebo, usually an "impure" one, as they often are. But it is not helpful to imply even indirectly that death can follow a pure placebo used in the usual fashion.

In *Placebos and the Philosophy of Medicine* Brody overinterprets a study of Lasagna:

Placebo reactions may resemble those of active drugs not only in the end results but also in the patterns of activity. These patterns include a peak effect a certain number of hours after administration of the drug, a cumulative effect of increase in symptom relief as the drug is continued over time, with a carryover effect after the drug is stopped, and a decrease in efficacy as the severity of the symptom increases.[21]

17. Bourne, H. R., The placebo: A poorly understood and neglected therapeutic agent, *Rational Drug Therapy* 5:1–5, 1971, quoted in Brody, *Placebos and the philosophy of medicine*.

18. Beecher, H. K., The powerful placebo, *JAMA* 159:1602–06, 1955.

19. Bok, S., *Lying*, New York: Pantheon, 1978, p. 165.

20. Kunin, C. M., Tupasi, T., and Craig, W. A., Use of antibiotics, *Ann. Intern. Med.* 79:555–60, 1973.

21. Lasagna, L., Laties, V. G., and Dohan, J. L., Further studies on the "pharmacology" of placebo administration, *J. Clin. Invest.* 37:533–37, 1958.

In fact Lasagna studied the effect of aspirin or a placebo on pain relief and the effect of a placebo given to patients with tuberculosis or chronic disease. In the latter study the patients were told that the tablets would increase their appetite and improve their "pep and energy." In both circumstances placebo therapy was associated with improvement which persisted beyond the time of administration. Moreover the investigators demonstrated a "peak effect" and a "cumulative effect," which looked like a pharmacologic study. They warned that such "pharmacological events would render interpretation of other drugs more difficult." But the point to remember is that they were studying pain and subjective phenomena, not objectively determined events. We should not carry the implication of their paper too far.

In evaluating the placebo response we must decide what we will evaluate. Is it objective disease or the diminution of complaints? Will we measure change in an organ's shape or size or a reduction in the patient's pain or suffering? The foregoing review suggests that it is by the relief of pain and suffering on a person-to-person level that we must assess the placebo effect. The placebo response may ameliorate diseases, but the evidence is not available, or at least I have not found it. We must keep firmly in mind the distinctions between the patient who has the disease and the disease itself. As Cassell has put it, echoing many others, "Doctors do not treat disease; they treat patients who have diseases."[22] It is the subjective improvement that we have to gauge.

Pain relief. Problems exist in the definition of pain relief. Pain relief in peptic ulcer, for example, has been defined in many different ways, even in controlled clinical trials: (1) the speed with which a single dose of antacid relieves a single attack, (2) the number of days of therapy required for complete relief of pain, (3) the number of pain-free days a patient may have in a week, (4) how often the patient is free of nocturnal pain, or (5) how many patients are pain-free at specific intervals after the start of therapy.[23] We must keep in mind the differences between the effects of a "dummy" placebo in a controlled clinical trial and the effects of placebo as gift and symbol.

Overall, placebos seem to relieve pain but not much else. But we have to look at what kinds of pain are relieved and in what circumstances. To do so it is important to classify pain in some kind of reasonable manner.

22. Cassell, E. J., The nature of suffering and the goals of medicine, *NEJM* 306: 637–45, 1982.
23. Gudjonson, B., and Spiro H. M., Response to placebos in ulcer disease, *Amer. J. Med.* 65:399–402, 1978.

Pain means different things to different people. It is not neatly tracked, and suffering, anxiety, and much more in the way of "central function" and assessment go to make up what is described as pain. To evaluate placebo responses we must go even further. Pain can be classified in different ways, as (1) acute or chronic, (2) mild or severe, (3) of known or unknown source, and (4) of limited or definite duration. It can of course also carry other characteristics.

There are so many ways to describe pain that it is not always easy to determine into which category pain that is relieved by placebo falls. Obviously the subject in a dental chair having his pain tolerance evaluated and manipulated by behavioral scientists knows that the pain is to be short-lived and worth enduring, since whatever was bothering him before will have been repaired, whereas the subject with a headache may wonder whether he has a brain tumor, and the subject with arm pain from an experimental heat lamp in the laboratory may have doubts about whether he should have volunteered for the study. Placebos will work differently in patients and in subjects depending upon several factors. But for now I am not interested in analyzing each kind of pain or in learning where and how such pain will be relieved by placebo. I call attention to the general phenomenon of pain and the importance of analyzing each study in terms of the kinds of pain and the circumstances in which it was evoked or relieved, and the kinds of people who had it.

Generally the pain of chronic disease has been studied for placebo benefit much more than that of acute disease. Much more needs to be done in this area. For example, in patients with acute localized muscle spasm, injections of saline into the painful area gave slightly more relief than a local anesthetic, but enough so that investigators wondered whether they were really performing acupuncture.[24]

The pain of angina pectoris is remarkably responsive to placebo, as Benson and McCallie recounted a few years ago. At first, in uncontrolled trials drug therapy for angina usually proves effective in 70 to 90 percent of patients, but gradually the number of people helped by a new drug diminishes to a 30 to 40 percent "placebo effectiveness."[25] Thirty to forty percent seems to be the baseline frequency with which pain is relieved by most placebos. Beecher calculated about a 35 percent baseline placebo effectiveness for all nonsurgical procedures in the 1960s.[26] In controlled clinical trials of duodenal ul-

24. Frost, F. A., Jessen, B., and Sigaard-Andersen, J., A control, double-blind comparison of mepivacaine injection versus saline injection for myofascial pain, *Lancet* 1:499–500, 1980.

25. Benson H., and McCallie D. P., Angina pectoris and the placebo effect, *NEJM* 300:1424–29, 1979.

26. Beecher, H. K., Surgery as placebo, *JAMA* 176:1102–07, 1961.

cer therapy, placebo effectiveness seldom falls below 35 or 45 percent, although it may rise as high as 60 percent or more depending upon the circumstances.

In the 1930s theophylline, at first, relieved pain of angina pectoris in about 76 percent of patients, but gradually proved to be no more effective than a placebo, helping only about 37 percent of patients, according to Benson and McCallie.[27] Khellin, at first touted as a remarkable discovery from Egypt, likewise finally proved no better than placebo. Since the same fate has befallen a number of other drugs touted for angina pectoris, controlled trials seem to be in order. But as Benson and McCallie conclude that even exercise tolerance is subject to the placebo effect, they discount the simple evaluation of such objective changes, without controlled trials, as evidence of effectiveness. In the past decade nitroglycerine patches applied to the chest over the heart have achieved enormous popularity for prolonged relief of angina pectoris. Levels of nitroglycerine were measured in the blood to reassure physicians that the patch was more than a poultice. Control trials with placebo, however, have "raised serious doubts about the clinical efficacy of these devices," which may have engendered only a strong placebo effect.[28]

Onset and Duration of Placebo Effect

The time in which placebos are reported to work is important. Within what time limit do we accept an event or change as a consequence of a placebo? The blood sugar level which falls an hour after a placebo is quite a different response from levels which return to normal over the six months of a control trial. Exactly what to ascribe to an intervention, when we are trying to separate mind-events from body-events, has bothered investigators since William James. How can I claim that a placebo affects only the person and not disease when I look at the 50 percent of patients whose ulcers heal on placebos in controlled trials? I argue that the placebo-dummy in those circumstances is given to act as a control for the passage of time, so that the beneficial relationship of being studied and cared for will not be mistaken for the effect of a drug. The placebo in those circumstances is given without intent to help. The placebo given by a doctor to a patient is given as an inactive drug, in the belief that it will be effective. But how many ulcers heal unseen, with no study? In general most studies suggest that if placebos work, they work quickly. Organic disease changes more slowly in response to therapy and it would be im-

27. Benson and McCallie, Angina pectoris and the placebo effect.
28. Parker, J. O., Efficacy of nitroglycerine patches: Fact or fancy? *Ann. Intern. Med.* 102:548–49, 1985.

possible, I suspect, to separate the natural history of a disease from any long-term benefit of a placebo, or a relationship between doctor and patient.

Studies of pain are the most pertinent, and they usually record an effect in minutes to hours. Many studies that are not laboratory controlled do not specify time intervals, but presumably observations extend over days and weeks. In the laboratory, Shapiro's study is representative.[29] He tried to measure the effect of a drug over the ensuing hour. If we are to take the endorphins as part of the mechanism of pain relief, then it seems reasonable to postulate that there may be a quick response and a slow response and that we may not be talking about the same thing when we refer to all such responses as the result of a placebo.

In clinical practice the clinician is usually talking about relief that is long-term, days or weeks rather than hours, but we must distinguish these effects if we are to wrest some sense out of the placebo response. One reason for part of the placebo effect may be statistical. Patients usually see physicians when their symptoms are at their worst; if the problem is a self-limited one, it may disappear a few days after the visit to the physician, who may then take credit for natural history.[30]

Placebos Improve Illness, Not Disease

My review, then, suggests that subjective complaints are helped a great deal, but that the evidence for objective improvement of diseases is not persuasive. George Bernard Shaw is said to have exclaimed at seeing the pile of crutches and eye glasses at the healing shrine of Lourdes, "But where are the wooden legs and glass eyes?" Again, it is important to keep in mind that we are not talking about the effects of a "dummy" placebo as in controlled clinical trials but rather about the effects of placebo as gift.

It seems reasonable to conclude that symptoms are what is helped in most collected series and that symptoms, by their very nature, must be "subjective" rather that "objective." For example, Haas lists analgesia, migraine, seasickness, rheumatism, dysmenorrhea, and other such complaints as yielding to placebo therapy.[31] Nowhere is there evidence that objective improvement in organic disease has occurred. Organic "disease" may indeed improve on placebo, but the reports are not available except as pain is relieved or ulcers disappear in con-

29. Shapiro, A. K., Struening, E. L., and Shapiro, E., The reliability and validity of a placebo test, *J. Psychiatr. Res.* 15:253–90, 1980.

30. Fields, H. L., Neurophysiology of pain and pain modulation, *Amer. J. Med.* 77(3A):2–8, 1984.

31. Haas, H., Fink, H., and Hartfeld, G., Das Placeboproblem, *Prog. Drug. Res.* 1:279–450, 1959.

trolled clinical trials. I have taken such cures or relief to come from the clinical situation, and not to stem from the placebo as such, but others may disagree. Warts, after all, do go away with all kinds of treatment.

In claiming that placebos affect persons and illness, not disease, I recognize the conceptual problems. The placebo could affect persons because of changes in neurotransmitters which then fill receptors to open or close channels, the brain modulating itself and in turn influencing disease. Fright can kill, voodoo can lead to sudden death, and malign influences can affect the normal person. People do "fight" cancer, die of fear, or keep going until "after the wedding," "until Christmas," or until they give up.

Moreover, high blood pressure, asthma, and many other disorders may be helped by suggestion, by placebo, and by many other nonspecific approaches. Yet for now, I put those in a "functional" rather than a disease category. We may show change in function, but I cannot find any evidence that we can show change in disease itself as measured by structure. I can take hopeful refuge in the notion that disease is multifactorial, that changing a patient's expectations may change his neurochemistry. Reducing stress, for example, may decrease the amount of catecholamines secreted and so diminish the likelihood of a cardiac arrhythmia. Asthma can be relieved by reassurance. Suggestion and consolation, hope and laughter, may well prove to have benefit for disease. I hope so. But for the dichotomies I have set up I have not found the evidence which I hope the future will bring.

In commenting on such problems, William James in 1890 concluded, "that a certain amount of brain physiology must be presupposed or included in Psychology. . . . Mental states occasion also changes in the calibre of blood vessels, or alteration in the heart beats, or processes more subtle still, in glands and viscera. If these are taken into account, as well as acts which follow at some *remote period* because the mental state was once there, it will be safe to lay down the general law that *no mental modification ever occurs which is not accompanied or followed by a bodily change.*"[32]

Neurobiological explorations make it possible to imagine that if emotions are programs in the brain, their currents can be influenced by words, by symbols, by the placebo. Neurobiology offers an explanation of how the placebo might work and consolation to physicians who demand mechanisms. All sensations change brain function: smell, taste, sight, hearing, touch are linked physiologically. The emotions seem likely to be a complex arrangement of brain function. If

32. James, W., The principles of psychology, vol. 1, New York: Dover, 1980, p. 5.

the emotions emerge hard-wired from the brain, words and symbols can have an effect on physiology, or even on disease, simply because we are constructed to receive them, our receptors await the right stimuli. The reaction to a disease could prove as substantial as the disease itself. For now, however, I draw the arbitrary division between disease and illness, fearing that in calling it arbitrary, I show myself a reductionist. Regardless of explanation, the observations on the placebo remain, and the course of action unchanged. Precisely because placebos help illness more than disease they are important to the doctor's understanding of his role and to our concepts of health and disease.

It may be pertinent to note that diseases can roughly be divided into three categories: (1) innocent, diseases that come and go quickly in which any intervention will appear to be helpful; (2) stubborn, that persist for some time and in which intervention of some variety is deemed helpful; and (3) most important, the intractable diseases that defy medical care yet need help. Physicians should demand proof of the disease that has been cured, especially if it seems to be relieved by apparently nonrational approaches.[33]

I have to conclude that relief comes with placebo, but that the evidence for placebo benefit for organic or structural biomedical disease is, to be complimentary, insubstantial. I have emphasized that physicians think of disease as what can be seen, measured, or photographed. The gratifying advances in the treatment and analysis of diseases have not been accompanied by equal advances in the management of pain and suffering, what we have agreed to call illness. Such illnesses probably represent 80 percent of most primary care doctors' practices, and it is that 80 percent which provides the people who might be helped by "alternative" medicine, Christian Science, placebo, and other approaches. They comprise a very large group indeed, and the help provided by "alternative" approaches is very important help regardless of the mechanisms involved.

In this conclusion I am supported by a study which looked at whether social and psychological factors in any way influenced survival of patients with many different cancers.[34] The authors of that paper concluded that the biology of the tumor overrode the "potential influence of life-style and psychosocial variables once the disease process is established." We would hope to the contrary, but as I have emphasized in this chapter, the evidence tells us otherwise.

33. Spiro, H. M., H2-blockers: How safe and how effective? *J. Clin. Gastroenterol.* 5(suppl.):143–47, 1983.

34. Cassileth, B. R., Lusk, E. J., Miller, D. S., et al., Psychosocial correlates of survival in advanced malignant disease? *NEJM* 312:1551–55, 1985.

What Kinds of Patients Respond to Placebo?

Approximately one-third of any group of people will prove in some way to be placebo responders, regardless of what they are being tested for. In controlled trials much effort is put into detecting such placebo responders and eliminating them as subjects. Getting rid of people who improve on placebo makes it easier to evaluate the benefit of a drug and sharpens statistical investigation. Yet when the drug is released for general use, such an approach overemphasizes the benefit of the drug for the general population, at least a third of whom might respond to a placebo. That is, if you get rid of placebo responders before you start your trial, you may get a more conclusive result. But when you later advertise your drug to doctors, they will give it to one-third of patients who might have been placebo responders.

For example, I have already recounted how controlled clinical trials of healing in peptic ulcer suggest that more than half the people getting a placebo benefit from the placebo. Their pain is relieved and their ulcers heal almost as fast as in the patients getting an active drug. Yet when the drug is released for general prescription, it is advertised for, and given to, most patients with peptic ulcer. The argument goes that physicians cannot predict the placebo responders and so must treat everyone, and I agree. But a case could be made for trying the weakest drug or even a placebo first. Sometimes what is feared to be only a placebo in the relief of pain turns out to have physiologic effect. Milk offers a good if parochial example (see chapter 4). Experiments remind us that we can only measure to the limits of our current technology. It is a mistake to take the results of any experiment as the whole explanation for a biological event. Milk may stimulate gastric acid by increasing calcium levels, as experiments a few years ago suggested, but future observations on endorphins and phospholipids may suggest why milk is still, paradoxically, so helpful.[35]

The Search for a Placebo Receptor Personality

Considerable work has gone into trying to predict the so-called placebo responder, to characterize them in terms of their (1) basic personality, (2) cultural and socioeconomic status, (3) suggestibility, or (4) their anxiety at the circumstances in which they find themselves. Most observers conclude that no specific personality characteristics have so far been proven. Shapiro has provided the review that most succeeding writers accept. Placebo reactors have been characterized as "compliant, religious, hypochondriac, anxious, as less educated and fre-

35. Spiro, H. M., Is milk so bad for the peptic ulcer patient? *J. Clin. Gastroenterol.* 3:219–20, 1981.

quently using cathartics; disturbed and likely to react to drugs with atypical reactions; anxious and depressed; dependent; ideational; neurotic; extroverted; and so on."[36]

Sex, age, and intelligence do not seem to matter. While the armchair observer might have predicted that suggestibility would have been important, no firm evidence supports the idea that the "suggestible" person is more likely to benefit from, or be affected by, a placebo.[37] Free-floating anxiety, particularly in patients with stress, seems to be the one factor that is most likely to be related to the likelihood of a placebo effect. Shapiro concludes that "there is no doubt left by a review of the literature that anxiety is an important element associated with placebo effects."[38]

Shapiro attempted to look at this question indirectly by "self-administered placebo tests" in which patients from a mental health clinic were given a placebo to take at home; after taking it, they were told to write down any effects of the "test medication." Coming to no firm answers from this study, he concluded that the placebo reaction was inconsistent and subject to unmeasurable variation, that a recognizable and reliable "placebo personality" did not exist, that measurement of the placebo response was really quite complicated, and finally that the "placebo test" as administered was an invalid measure of the placebo effect.

Later, in 1980, Shapiro was still trying to devise a placebo test which would predict who might respond to a placebo.[39] Depressed and anxious psychiatric outpatients were given a "green capsule" which was a placebo. They were asked to note their symptoms over the next hour; control patients were simply told "to spend the next hours in a quiet room to see how your symptoms spontaneously vary." The Cornell group made extensive statistical analyses, and concluded:

> Thus, patients react differently according to whether pre-placebo symptoms are absent or present and whether they receive a therapeutic stimulus or a non-therapeutic stimulus. A possible interpretation of these data is that patients without pre-placebo symptoms have nothing or little to feel better about, and may feel worse if given something they don't need, whether it is a therapeutic or a non-therapeutic stimulus. Patients with low levels of pre-placebo symptoms improve with any type of stimulus, whether it is a tangi-

36. Shapiro, A. K., The placebo response, in *Modern perspectives in world psychiatry*, vol. 2, ed. J. E. Howells, Edinburgh: Oliver and Boyd, 1971.

37. Buckalew, L. W., Ross, S., Starr, J. L., Nonspecific factors in drug effects: Placebo personality, *Psychological Reports* 48:3−8, 1981.

38. Shapiro, The placebo response.

39. Shapiro, Struening, and Shapiro, The reliability and validity of a placebo test.

ble therapeutic drug stimulus or an intangible non-therapeutic stimulus. However, patients with higher levels of pre-placebo symptoms feel worse than before if given nothing and feel better if given a therapeutic stimulus. The therapeutic stimulus seems to protect patients from increased symptomatic discomfort.

Not everyone agrees with Shapiro's conclusions. Analyzing studies from the psychological perspective, Jospe concludes:

> Our overall picture of the placebo reactors is that they are people who depend upon, and trust in, other people's ability to help them. ... (p. 90)
>
> The placebo reactors place much reliance on others to be the agents in their therapeutic change. . . . They cannot get along well without other people, even though at times they allow themselves to be dominated by others, especially authority figures (like physicians). The research in acquiescence has been so impressive that further research on the role of this characteristic in the placebo responder would undoubtedly yield very fruitful results.[40]

One study which supports the importance of "acquiescence" showed that college students who were psychiatric outpatients because of anxiety and depression improved on a placebo over a period of seven days.[41] The authors felt that improvement was related as much to yea-saying as to anything else. As I have generally ignored the overwhelming literature on placebo response in psychotherapy, I call attention to this observation.

Brody questions whether there is a "single personality type" that characterizes the placebo reactor even though he is optimistic about the possibility that the non-reactor can be more clearly defined.[42] I agree with Brody's conclusion that it would be more fruitful to look at the "entire placebo context" rather than at the placebo reactor.

Clinicians recognize the anxious person who needs help as the prototypical patient who might benefit from a placebo. It has been suggested that the more severe the pain, the greater the likelihood of a placebo analgesic response, but while this proved true of patients with dental pain, it did not prove quite so possible to demonstrate the same improvement in patients with psychoneurotic "somatization." So-called autonomic awareness, the awareness of such bodily functions as heart rate, digestion, or respiration, is an ill-defined measurement which sounds as if it ought to have some bearing on the placebo response but which apparently does not.

40. Jospe, *The placebo effect*.
41. McNair, D. M., Gardos, F., Haskell, D. S., et al., Placebo response, placebo effect, and two attributes, *Psychopharmacology* 63:245–50, 1979.
42. Brody, *Placebos and the philosophy of medicine*.

Nonreactors have been defined as "more rigid and emotionally controlled." Shapiro suggests, indeed, that his own preliminary study "indicates that non-reactors are rigid, authoritarian, stereotypic, tend to use the mechanism of denial, and are not psychologically oriented. . . . Negative reactors rely more on inner stimuli, and tend to have more paranoid and masochistic traits."[43] The reader may turn to Jospe's 1978 book for a painstaking and critical review of the behavioral investigations into the placebo. Jospe concludes his study of the placebo reaction with an important caution: "Such research, and in fact any research on the placebo effect, should not be conducted with non-patients. Laboratory experiments are not clinical situations. . . . An experimenter is not a therapist, a subject is not a patient, and a laboratory is not a clinic."[44] Such cautionary advice is borne out by recent work which shows that the endogenous opioid analgesic mechanisms are more likely to be stimulated by intense pain stimuli than by short mild stimuli.[45]

Informing the Patient

The literature is sparse on the effect of a placebo given to a patient who is told that he is getting a placebo. Park and Covi, in a much-quoted study in the 1960s, did just that for fifteen "newly admitted neurotics."[46] After an initial evaluation of one hour, they told these patients, "Many people with your kind of condition have also been helped by what are sometimes called 'sugar pills', and we feel that a so-called sugar pill may help you, too. Do you know what a sugar pill is? A sugar pill is a pill with no medicine in it at all. I think this pill will help you as it has helped so many others. Are you willing to try this pill?"

One week later, thirteen of fourteen patients who took the pills reported improvement, and overall there was a 41 percent decrease in symptoms. Of course there are special problems in generalizing from this study of "neurotic" patients. They had already undergone a one-hour interview, which presumably brought its own benefits, and there was no control trial of either drug or interview. Recognizing these problems, the authors admitted that they were not sure whether the placebo treatment they gave "could be viewed as having some affinity to psychotherapy" or simply, in agreement with others, that it was

43. Shapiro, The placebo response.

44. Jospe, *The placebo effect.*

45. Fields, H. L., and Levine, J. D., Biology of placebo analgesia, *Amer. J. Med.* 70:745–46, 1981.

46. Park, L. C., and Covi, L., Nonblind placebo trial: An exploration of neurotic outpatients' responses to placebo when its inert content is disclosed, *Arch. Gen. Psychiatr.* 12:336–45, 1965.

"produced by the patients' faith in the efficacy of the therapist and his technique." But this important study suggests that placebos can work even when patients are told the truth about what they are getting.

Physiological Effects

It is important to distinguish between physiological effects which have been reported in normal subjects after placebo administration and the improvement in symptoms or complaints in patients who are—let us not forget—sick or in pain. For example, although nausea, sleepiness, or other complaints may be engendered by placebo in normal subjects, that is quite different from the events in the sick person. The intent of the investigator is quite different from the intent of the clinician. I do not know of any studies of pathophysiological changes in the sick person given a placebo for healing and not as part of a clinical trial.

I wonder whether we really can compare the effect of a placebo on normal physiology to the effect of a placebo on pathophysiology of disease. Presumably in normal subjects emotions can influence normal physiological activities. For example, gastric secretion which is not already increased under the influence of some pathologic force probably does increase when someone is angry or anxious. Yet when an ulcer is present, other forces may drive the pathophysiology so predominantly as to submerge any observable effect of placebo. Anger at being given an injection could have changed, indeed did change, Tom's gastric secretion in the Cornell experiments. But the evidence that the gastric secretion of the duodenal ulcer patient is similarly affected is far less persuasive. Strong emotions surely affect diseases, but we need better evidence that the kind of "soft" emotions engendered by the placebo have any effect on physiology in disease as well as in health.

The material is too complex for current assessment. Common sense might tell us that the person with a dependent personality, with faith in others and particularly in physicians, is more likely to be relieved—in current parlance, to generate his own endorphins— than someone who is withdrawn and skeptical. Or at least that the acquiescent person, anxious to please, will convince himself that he has less pain and so report it in a way he might not do if he were sitting at home taking a pill all alone. Confusion between patient and subject, and between clinical situation and research setting, makes it hard to conclude that the placebo reactor personality has, so far at least, been well defined, or that it can even be defined.

I suspect that almost everyone can respond to a placebo, regardless of education or culture or most of the other determinants so assiduously studied, in the right circumstances. Not everyone does respond to a placebo, of course. Studies in the laboratory suggest that overall about 35 percent of persons do so respond, but it is difficult or impossible to characterize them ahead of time. In some studies the number is higher, but the question which deserves an answer is why do not all people respond, especially if the mechanisms are in place in the neuroendocrine analgesic systems? What is there about some people that makes them good placebo responders? Fields and Levine have reviewed evidence pointing to the inconsistency of the placebo response in any one person: a woman might respond with relief of post partum or ischemic pain on one occasion, but not on the next.[47]

Some years ago in Cincinnati, medical students were given placebo pills after they had been told only that they were to receive either stimulant or sedative drugs and what the stimulant or sedative effects might be. They were then given either one or two pink or blue capsules without further information; they did not know that the color and number of capsules differed from subject to subject. Thirty percent of the subjects noticed drug-induced changes; on the whole sedative responses occurred six times more frequently than stimulant ones. Blue capsules were more likely to produce sedative effects than the pink ones, and students taking two capsules were more likely to report severe effects.[48]

The suggestibility of sophisticated if anxious medical students reminds us of how careful we must be about placebo responses. Circumstances will vary, and the reversion to a helpless infantile state when people get sick surely must enhance the likelihood of a placebo effect. The placebo response is greatest when there is the most anxiety, and when pain is severe. But few of us will not be helped by a placebo at some time or other. I take the response to a placebo as a testimony to our common humanity, to most people's need for community and a friend in time of troubles. Most men and women are not lone wolves.

47. Fields and Levine, Biology and placebo analgesia.
48. Blackwell, B., Bloomfield, S. S., and Buncher, C. R., Demonstration to medical students of placebo responses and non-drug factors, *Lancet* 1:1279–82, 1972.

7
Patients and Pain

The foregoing review suggests that symptoms are relieved by placebos, but diseases biomedically defined remain unchanged except insofar as they were getting better on their own. Pain is paramount among the complaints which are relieved by a placebo and relief of pain is one of the common reasons for patients to seek out doctors. Pain has been defined by an official body dedicated to its study as "an unpleasant sensory and emotional experience associated with actual or potential tissue damage or described in terms of such damage."[1]

For the clinician, pain needs no definition beyond an operational one: "I am in pain," or "I have pain." It is important, therefore, to review some pertinent aspects of the physiology of pain perception. In the discussion which follows, I will not distinguish between acute and chronic pain. The division between them lies at six months, a major distinction being the absence of physical findings in the patient with chronic pain in contrast to the objective evidence found in the patient with acute pain. Instead I will focus on more general concepts which may provide some clues about how the placebo response works.

THE PAIN PATIENT

The patient with chronic pain casts the problems into sharp relief. Practitioners know implicitly how important is the patient himself in determining the response to a disease or injury, and how much a problem will disable him. One person will keep working with a bad

1. IASP Subcommittee on Taxonomy Pain Terms, *Pain* 6:249–52, 1979.

cold that will put another to bed for a week. Hypochondriacs are well known to laymen and physicians alike; such chronic invalids are not new. The Greeks knew them. In *The Republic,* Plato speaks of a physician, Herodicus, who

> by a combination of training and doctoring found out a way of torturing first and chiefly himself, and secondly the rest of the world . . . by the invention of lingering death; for he had a mortal disease which he perpetually tended, and as recovery was out of the question, he passed his entire life as a valetudinarian; he could do nothing but attend upon himself, and he was in constant torment whenever he departed in anything from his usual regimen, and so dying hard, by the help of science he struggled on to old age.[2]

The apparently healthy patient wrapped up in his pain which defies explanation and investigation is surely different from the patient with pain from pancreatic cancer, as severe as any pain can be, who persists in his work and in his life. People perceive and interpret pain in different ways, not all of which are susceptible to a simple neurological interpretation,[3] even when they have cancer.[4] The physician may learn about disease, detecting and evaluating it objectively, but it is the patient who knows his pain and interprets it.[5]

Pain is not wholly bad. Hart reminds us that pain can be a friend because it calls attention to disorders that demand treatment: "The patient with a chronic pain that cannot be shaken off has to learn to live with it and to evolve spiritual complexities to make it tolerable. . . . Relatively few patients with chronic pains ask their physician for death and deliverance, and very few commit suicide."[6] These "little martyrs," as Hart calls them, stand in contrast to the patients for whom pain is a career, a way of life. For these pain patients, as Hart puts it, "Pain is spelt with a capital letter and is truly an old friend. . . . This is not a medical or psychiatric problem, but a social one that concerns the personality. Here the Pain is not just an old friend but an essential part of the sufferer's existence: it is not so much a part of, as a partner in, the suffer's life."

Fundamentally, most physicians recognize how different can be the responses to pain regardless of whether it has a detectable origin or is psychogenic. In *The Puzzle of Pain* Melzack comments:

2. Plato, *The Republic,* New York: Scribner's Sons, 1928, book 3, p. 121.
3. Addison, R. G., Chronic pain syndrome, *Amer. J. Med.* 77(3A):54–58, 1984.
4. Foley, K. M., The treatment of cancer pain, *NEJM* 313:84–95, 1985.
5. Spiro, H. M., Pain and perfectionism, *NEJM* 294:829–30, 1976; Posner, R. B., Physician-patient communication, *Am. J. Med.* 77(3A):59–64, 1984.
6. Hart, F. D., Pain as an old friend, *Brit. Med. J.* 1:1405–07, 1979.

Pain, we now believe, refers to a category of complex experiences, not to a specific sensation that varies only along a single intensity dimension. The word "pain," in this formulation, is a linguistic label that categorizes an endless variety of qualities. (p. 41)

Pain is not a single quality of experience that can be specified in terms of defined stimulus conditions. It may be agreed that pain, like vision and hearing, is a complex perceptual experience. (pp. 45–46)

The psychological evidence strongly supports the view of pain as a perceptual experience as quality and intensity are influenced by the unique past history of the individual, by the meaning he gives to the pain producing situation and by his "state of mind" at the moment. . . . In this way pain becomes a function of the whole individual, including his present thoughts and fears as well as his hopes for the future. (pp. 47–48)[7]

PAIN AND CULTURE

Physicians also know that people from different traditions deal with their pains and aches in sometimes dramatically different ways. Melzack comments on couvade in this context:

There is much evidence that pain is not simply a function of the amount of bodily damage alone. Rather, the amount and quality of pain we feel are also determined by our previous experiences and how well we remember them, by our ability to understand the causes of the pain and to grasp its consequences. Even the culture in which we have been brought up plays an essential role in how we feel and respond to pain. (p. 21)

In some societies the husband of a pregnant woman gets into bed and groans with pain while the woman, altogether unconcerned, bears the baby. Cultural backgrounds have well-known influences on the pain perception threshold; for example, people of Mediterranean origin report feeling pain at levels of radiant heat that Northern Europeans describe only as warm.[8] In some studies in the 1950s, presumably now archaic, "Old Americans" proved more stoical in reac-

7. Melzack, R., *The puzzle of pain*, New York: Basic, 1973.
8. Wolff, B. B., and Langley, F., Culture and pain, *Amer. Anthropol.* 70:494–501, 1968; Wolff, B. B., Ethocultural factors influencing pain and illness behavior, *Clin. J. Pain* 1:23–80, 1985.

tion to pain than Jews or Italians. Jews wanted to know what caused the pain, whereas Italians were satisfied with its relief.[9]

In addition to cultural factors and past experience of pain, the meaning of the situation, how much attention is paid to it, anxiety, and suggestion are all important in determining how much pain someone feels as well as how he responds to the pain.[10] For example, the reaction to picking up a very hot cup may be different when the cup is paper and we are at a football game than when it is a china cup in someone's living room.[11]

Pain Relief Systems

There are two logically distinct but interwoven systems which relieve pain: (1) a neurological network, highly organized and complex; and (2) a hormonal supply of endogenous opiates which permeates the body.[12] As more is learned about neurotransmitters and the neuroendocrine apparatus, the interrelated unified nature of neural and hormonal systems should become apparent, but at the moment it is convenient to think of them as separate but equal.

Neurological control of pain. The central nervous network monitors, perceives, and changes the perception of pain. Feeling pain is more than a single stimulus-response reaction suggested by the now-outmoded specificity theory. For many physicians, however, pain remains only a simple response to a specific stimulus. In medical school they may have learned more sophisticated theory, but from working with physicians of all ages and training for over thirty-five years, I am convinced that when physicians see a patient complaining of pain in the arm, belly, or elsewhere, most of them look for a single point source so that a single therapeutic intervention will be appropriate. Consciously or unconsciously, practicing physicians are still strongly influenced by the outmoded specificity theory, which held that a specific receptor in the skin—a pain receptor—responds to a painful stimulus to send messages by way of nerve fibers, to a pain center in the brain. A one-to-one relationship between receptor type, fiber size, and the kind of painful stimulus (cutting, burning, and so forth) in a

9. Zborowski, M., Cultural components in responses to pain, *J. Soc. Issues* 8:16–30, 1952.

10. Engel, G. L., "Psychogenic" pain and the pain-prone patient, *Amer. J. Med.* 26:899–918, 1959.

11. Mechanic, D., Social psychological factors affecting the presentation of bodily complaints, *NEJM* 286:1131–39, 1972.

12. Levine, J., Pain and analgesia: The outlook for more rational treatment, *Ann. Intern. Med.* 100:269–76, 1984; Thompson, J. W., Opioid peptides, *Brit. Med. J.* 1:259–60, 1984.

fixed stimulus-response relationship seems congenially simple: The more intense the stimulus, the greater the pain. Unfortunately the notion is incorrect. The theory has influenced medical notions of pain as a "fixed, straight-through conceptual nervous system" for so long, however, that it seems almost intuitively accepted by physicians who know about the gate theory, about endorphins, and even about the paramount influence the higher brain centers have on the perception of pain.

The gate theory. H. R. Marshall, so Melzack tells us,[13] was the first to emphasize that pain is more than just a sensation we feel. Pain has a strong affective quality; how we feel about the pain may be as important as how we feel that pain or its objective intensity. Painful stimuli *simultaneously* influence both sensory processes and affective emotional processes. Unfortunately Marshall's theory, which is a forerunner of present ideas, was ignored for many years in favor of the specificity theory and observations which suggested that pain fibers led directly to the pain center and that only *after* the pain was felt could it be evaluated, perceived, and appropriate action taken.

Large and small nerves. Noordenbos provided the basis for modern concepts of pain mechanisms.[14] He found that small nerve fibers carried pain impulses, but that pain perception could be inhibited by impulses from larger nerve fibers which ran alongside the small nerves. The small nerve fibers, so-called *C-fibers* which account for pain perception, can be activated by many stimuli, from heat to the chemical mediators of inflammation; the more repeated the stimuli, the lower the threshold for pain perception.

Germane to placebo action are the large-diameter non-nociceptive nerve fibers which act as the gate to inhibit the perceptual pain. These large fibers do not carry pain messages and, hence, are called non-nociceptive. They simply inhibit pain transmission at the level of the spinal cord. Fields suggests that stimulation of these fibers explains the effectiveness of massage and acupuncture.[15]

Modern neurological studies which supplement the gate control theory, emphasize the complexity of pain sensations, to enable us to begin to glimpse the mechanisms by which the placebo might influence pain perception, the affective or emotional state.[16]

13. Melzack, *The puzzle of pain.*
14. Noordenbos, W., *Pain,* Amsterdam: Elsevier, 1959.
15. Fields, H. L., Neurophysiology of pain and pain modulation, *Amer. J. Med.* 77(3A):2–8, 1984.
16. Ibid.; Sternbach, R. A., *The psychology of pain,* New York: Raven, 1978.

In addition, the sympathetic nervous system has some role in pain perception, but the exact mechanism by which distortion of sympathetic nerves leads to the unpleasant sensations called *causalgia* need not concern us now. Secretion of catecholamines, especially serotonin, seems to be important and may underline the explanation of why tricyclic antidepressants are also such effective pain relievers. For Fields, they represent a "totally new class of centrally acting non-addicting pain killers."[17]

Modulation of pain. Basically, the gate-control theory suggests that a mechanism in the dorsal horns of the spinal cord acts like a gate, increasing or decreasing the flow of impulses from peripheral fibers to the central nervous system.[18] Running from the large-diameter fibers, which inhibit pain by closing or lowering the gate, pathways lead to a central control area in the upper brain which in turn influences, through descending fibers, the "modulating properties of the spinal gating mechanism." This central control trigger may open or close the gate, raising or lowering the threshold for pain once signals from the body have been identified and evaluated. The important point is that the gate is raised or lowered "in terms of prior experience" *before* the action system responsible for pain perception and response is activated. This mechanism Melzack calls the "central biasing mechanism":

> The gate control theory also suggests that psychological processes such as past experience, attention, and emotion may influence pain perception and response by acting on the spinal gating mechanism. Some of these psychological activities may open the gate while others may close it. (p. 71)

Stimulation of discrete sites in the brain raises the threshold at which animals and humans can feel pain. Thus it is that pain can be controlled by modulation of the input. It has a sensory component depending upon the intensity of the stimulus, but it also has a very important affective individual component. Whether the input is local or cortical may depend on such individual reaction. Many psychological processes influence pain and with the gate theory there is at least a physiological concept for recognizing how placebos may work.

We must distinguish between *pain threshold,* which is the intensity of the noxious stimulus necessary for a person to perceive pain, and *pain tolerance,* the duration of time or intensity at which a person accepts a stimulus before recognizing it, or responding to it, (or maybe just telling us about it) as pain. Beecher may be quoted in this regard: "The

17. Fields, Neurophysiology of pain.
18. Melzack, *The puzzle of pain;* Thompson, Opioid peptides.

great power of the placebo provides one of the strongest supports for the view that drugs that are capable of altering subjective responses and symptoms do so to an important degree through their effect on the reaction component of suffering."[19]

The Endogenous Analgesia System

The body maintains a constant state as best it can. In health the constituents of the blood such as the level of sugar or electrolytes are kept within a very narrow range. When disease alters these constituents, mechanisms come into play to try to return them toward normal. For example, when the sodium level of the blood is depleted, the healthy kidney stops excreting sodium until the normal level is restored. Fever is a therapeutic defense against infection; but even so, fever stimulates mechanisms which try to bring the body temperature back to normal. It seems to be a general rule that after any injury, the body will try to restore matters to normal, using feedback controls to tell when to stop.

It should come as no surprise, then, that pain also triggers a system for its own relief. It makes sense to think of severe pain as stimulating endogenous analgesic systems and even that pain neutralizes those systems once they are activated. Though it may not be justified by current knowledge, I think of morphine as relieving pain, and I think of pain as counteracting the effects of too much morphine. That could be why people who have taken an overdose of a sedative are kept awake and walked around, at least by the laity who can do little more. Wakefulness may be the physiological antidote to sedation just as pain could be the physiological antidote to analgesia.

Opiate is a well-known term which refers specifically to any product of the opium poppy. The effect of most such naturally occurring products are counteracted in the body by *naloxone*, which has proven a remarkably helpful antidote to narcotic overdosage. *Opioid* is the term derived from opiate to refer to any compound, natural or synthetic, which has an effect which can be antagonized in the body by naloxone.

There are five groups of naturally occurring opioid peptides: (1) enkephalins, (2) dynorphins, (3) endorphins, (4) peptides from body fluids such as milk, and (5) "others."[20] Opioid peptides inhibit the neurotransmission of pain acting either as (1) short-acting neurotransmitters or (2) long-acting neural hormones. How they work is not completely within our current grasp, and a knowledge of where they work is not essential to understanding possible placebo mechanisms. It is enough to know that there are naturally occurring opioid

19. Beecher, H. K., The powerful placebo, *JAMA* 159:1602–06, 1955.
20. Thompson, Opioid peptides.

receptors in the brain, gut, and elsewhere. Opioids and opiates generated endogenously or given by mouth or by injection fit into receptors to activate pain relief systems. In some ways it is fortunate that pain above a certain intensity is required to stimulate the endogenous opiate systems that remain inactive in normal physiological circumstances. Short-duration, low-intensity stimuli (mild pain) are less effective in getting the system going than longer, continued, more intense pain. This makes sense because pain is a warning system, and one which made us ignore a hot stove, for example, would be more harmful than helpful.

Just how all this new knowledge will ultimately influence understanding of placebo analgesia is hard to predict. The simplest position holds that placebos will prove to stimulate endogenous endorphins or enkephalins, by way of the mind or by learned conditioned responses. Once the investigator can measure the strength of the placebo response by the level of endorphins generated, he can then characterize the circumstances and stimuli which activate the response and begin to quantitate the placebo response. Then we will be much further along in understanding the mechanisms of the placebo response, so that we can deal with it rationally.

But matters are not yet that advanced. And if they were, if we could measure endorphins accurately, we might still find much that was not understood. For example, a blue pill might turn out to stimulate a higher level of endorphins than a red one, getting a pill in the hospital might be more productive of higher enkephalin levels than buying one in a drug store, and so forth. Still, the mystery of why one person can so affect another is one that we can already examine, although we cannot measure how it happens. The mystery of the placebo will still be with us even as we spend many years trying to understand and to quantitate the placebo response. Leibnitz was the first to suggest that if we could stroll through a very large brain, looking at all its circuits, we would still not understand where love or hope or faith resided. The reductionist will counter that on such a stroll we would see the circuits moving and might have a clearer idea, but I think that is a long time off, despite the mapping of the brain of a small worm.

As it happens, conclusions are in conflict because there are no current accurate techniques for measuring the opioid analgesic systems. Some studies suggest that placebos stimulate endorphins and others that they do not because they rely upon indirect assessments of placebo analgesia by naloxone. For example, observers studying dental pain have found that patients who respond to a placebo will have more pain if they are given naloxone, a substance which inhibits endorphin activity.[21] In contrast naloxone has no such effect in patients whose pain has not responded to a placebo. In general observers have been taking the worsening of pain by naloxone to implicate endorphin relief of pain,[22] but it is so indirect a measure that understanding will improve when endorphins can be measured directly.

In the meantime Levine suggests that placebos can be divided into two physiological categories, inactive and active.[23] He suggests that an inactive placebo has no direct physiological action whereas an active placebo produces a physiological or pharmacological clue, such as an increase in pain which then activates one of the endogenous mechanisms. We will still have to find room for the nonopioid mechanisms as well: stress makes some people feel pain more readily and makes others ignore it. Such observations will have to be fit into the system. Then, how will we explain how that "inactive" placebo works?

At any rate current understanding suggests that there are at least three mechanisms for endogenous pain relief. Two are neurological and one is hormonal, but the more that is learned about neurotransmitters and neuropeptides, the more such a division seems artificial, because (1) areas in the brain inhibit pain perception by way of descending pathways that control what information reaches the brain; (2) neural circuits in the spinal column inhibit pain transmission locally, a local gating mechanism which in part must be responsible for relief by acupuncture or counterirritants; (3) the third mechanism, only recently begun to be explored, is comprised of the opioid circuits; (4) there may well be a fourth mechanism, a nonopioid pain-relieving system, related to the sympathetic nervous system to the catecholamines, and even to gastrointestinal-brain hormones such as cholecystokinin.[24]

Relief of pain by drugs can come in different ways: (1) the transmission of pain can be blocked; (2) mechanisms to suppress pain can be stimulated; or (3) drugs can make patients indifferent to pain. Drugs like aspirin, acetaminophen, or the nonsteroidal anti-inflammatory agents, block transmission peripherally. In contrast opiates

21. Grevert, P., Albert, L. H., and Goldstein, A., Partial antagonism of placebo analgesia by naloxone, *Pain* 16:129–43, 1983.

22. Beecher, The powerful placebo; Grevert, Albert, and Goldstein, Partial antagonism.

23. Levine, Pain and analgesia.

24. Graceley, R. H., Dubner, R., Wolsker, P. J., et al., Placebo and naloxone can alter post-surgical pain by separate mechanisms, *Nature* 306:264–65, 1983; Stacher, G., Steinringer, H., Schmieres, G., et al., Ceruletide increases dose dependently both jejunal motor activity and threshold and tolerance to experimentally induced pain in healthy man, *Gut* 25:513–19, 1984.

such as morphine or codeine act centrally on the brain to activate the pain-suppression mechanism. It is becoming customary to refer to such pain-relieving agents by the supposed locus of their action, as central or peripheral analgesics.

The mechanisms of placebo analgesia are complex. Kirsch makes the observation that it would be more profitable to view endorphin release as an effect of placebos rather than as a cause of placebo.[25] Current studies are important because they will begin to give an idea of what is and what is not known and may someday make it possible to characterize the healing personality, for example. But will knowing that one physician stimulates more endorphins than another explain why that physician is more effective? That one patient generates more endorphins than another? Will measurements do more than help us glimpse the mechanism? Understanding the mechanisms will not help very much in understanding how, for whom, and if the placebo works. Do we not already know the remarkable feature, the triumph of the placebo, that one person can help another simply by trying?

25. Kirsch, I., Response expectancy as a determinant of experience and behavior, *American Psychologist* 40:1189–1202, 1985.

8

Autonomy and Responsibility: Some Famous Patients

T his chapter examines the stories of Norman Cousins and Franz Ingelfinger, accounts which lie at opposite ends of a spectrum.[1] Cousins celebrates the power of the person to heal himself, with an acquiescent doctor in the background, while Ingelfinger relates the peace which came from turning over his problems to someone else. Dr. Franz Ingelfinger knew too much; he was one of the world's experts in the disease that struck him. Norman Cousins did not know enough and ploughed on, confident in his quasi-knowledge. Ingelfinger was the editor of the *New England Journal of Medicine* who opened its pages for Cousins's first report. Ingelfinger's own story was published after his death in that same journal. Although these writers are linked, their lessons are different.

NORMAN COUSINS'S STORY

In 1976 Norman Cousins gained wide notice with the story of his 1964 illness—a story that might have seemed as unfathomable to the physician as the casting-out of devils, had it not been published in the *New England Journal of Medicine*. Because of that journal's general prestige, Cousins's account was widely accepted by people anxious for a clue to self-help and physicians overly guilty about their technological emphasis and prowess.

The Complaint

In August 1964 Cousins developed general achiness and gradually increasing difficulty moving his neck, arms, hands, fingers, and legs.

1. Cousins, N., Anatomy of an illness (as perceived by the patient), *NEJM* 295: 1458–63, 1976; Inglefinger, F. J., Arrogance. *NEJM* 1507–11, 1980.

During a very trying hospital admission he writes that there was "no agreement on a precise diagnosis," even if there was "a general consensus" that he had "a serious collagen illness." Experts suggested the diagnosis of ankylosing spondylitis and one of them told Cousins's physician that he had "one chance in 500" of full recovery. We are not given the evidence on which these diagnoses were based and must consider them as conjectural as those of a witch doctor without data. With so lugubrious a prospect, Cousins got involved in his own care enough to convince his physician to give him vitamin C intravenously in doses "far enough beyond any recorded dose."

The rest of the story has become a medical classic. To encourage his will to live and the "full exercise of the affirmative emotions," Cousins moved out of the hospital into a hotel and arranged for old movies and video tapes to be shown to him. "Belly-laughter" proved helpful. Cousins and his physician were convinced, so the story goes, that laughter had a salutary effect on his body's chemistry. At the end of several weeks of ascorbic acid and laughter, a "remission" was achieved.

This aspect of Cousins's case suggests the difference between rational medicine and the irrational approach which so dismays the physician thinking about placebo. Although Cousins improved, there is no evidence of a cause-and-effect relation between "therapy" and cure. The kinds of reasons Cousins brought for his therapy are the kinds of partial explanations seized upon by celebrated nutritionists and other popular therapists, a kind of specific celebration of a possible effect abstracted from a general view. We can always find a reason to do something.

Kahn puts it well:

> From a profusion of guesses, influences, suppositions, hypotheses, possibilities, speculations, Cousins, by idiosyncratic alignment and juxtaposition, has chosen allergy, adrenal exhaustion, red blood cell clumping, placebo effect, endorphins, Vitamin C, cell oxidation, unknown biochemical effects of the pituitary stimulated by mental processes, etc., to erect a structure that is only one of the several score he could have created just as easily and with equal validity from the same building blocks. . . . We enter the realm of scientism, the use of scientific terminology and data for unscientific purposes, the artificial and arbitrary linear linkage of scientific material to support unjustified conclusions.[2]

2. Kahn, S., The anatomy of Norman Cousins' illness, *Mt. Sinai J. Med.* 48:305–14, 1981.

Professional Responsibility

Cloaked in rationality and late twentieth-century science, the thesis is not dissimilar from the reasoning behind many nineteenth-century panaceas. Twentieth-century charlatans also plunder philosophy to supply a reason for their treatments, and it is this simulation of science which enrages physicians. It would be hard for a licensed physician to justify such measures for another patient without more precise marshalling of evidence of potential injury and benefit. It is all right for my wife, a schoolteacher, to suggest as large doses of vitamin C to her friends as she gives to me. As a professional I have to weigh the evidence. Whether Cousins's physician went too far in allowing his prominent friend to decide upon such therapy must be asked. If Cousins had worked out a rational scheme to show that cutting off a finger might cure him and if Cousins had felt strongly enough to insist upon that, would his physician have agreed? Psychiatrists do talk of a patient who feared that she would be impregnated by the Holy Spirit and whose delusions were cured by hysterectomy. Such episodes remind us of the frailty of medical decision-making. Presumably, Cousins's physician decided that vitamin C intravenously was harmless, that the outlook was grim in any case, and what followed was a happy outcome. But we do not know whether the effect represents placebo effect, natural history, or a pharmacological benefit which demands further study.

Physicians have questioned whether Cousins had any serious chronic disease or whether his illness was a self-limited one which would have disappeared with any therapy. They have really no way of knowing, for no objective account has been published, as far as I know. I wrote to Mr. Cousins asking for some objective data from his physician. He graciously sent me an inscribed copy of the book which grew from his article, but I did not find any relevant objective data there.[3] I wrote to his physician, but my letter was returned. I have to conclude that the most famous case of self-help in the 1970s remains simply an account by a patient whose beliefs have been widely promulgated and who has had an enormous (and beneficial) influence on opinion simply because of his prominence. Indeed he now holds an appointment at UCLA Medical School and was made an honorary M.D. by the New Haven County Medical Association at its two hundredth anniversary. But I do not know how to interpret his report except as an example of a man escaping from the frustrations of his

3. Cousins, N., *Anatomy of an illness as perceived by the patient,* New York: Bantam, 1979.

physicians in the hospital and allowing the natural course of events to go unimpeded by medicine. To be sure, had he stayed in the hospital, he might have undergone more diagnostic maneuvers and received several other drugs with their myriad effects—and side effects.

As Ruderman puts it, "And this may, very often, be the value of the 'placebo': it frees the patient from other standard or experimental drugs, which may overwhelm the body's defences, or create diseases of their own—whose harmful effects may be greater than their benefits."[4]

He was probably lucky to leave. Like most other physicians, I have to conclude that he got better on his own while the movies beguiled him into passing time, but that the laughter alone did not cure him.

Despite these reservations, I applaud Cousins's conclusions and the skill with which he has raised important questions. I simply disagree with his premises. Most physicians reading the account probably believe, as Cousins himself fully recognizes, that he was "probably the beneficiary of a mammoth venture in self-administered placebos." This is a hypothesis which he does not disregard, but Cousins asks a very important question; "Is it possible that love, hope, faith, laughter, confidence, and the will to live have therapeutic value?" In *The Healing Heart* Cousins suggests, properly, that "laughter was just a metaphor for the entire range of the positive emotions" (p. 50). But he clearly has second thoughts: "I never regarded the positive emotions, however, as a substitute for scientific treatment. I saw them as providing an auspicious environment for medical care."[5] Yet I cannot see that in that first recorded illness he received standard or rational medical care.

Miller echoes him: "To what extent do laughter, beauty, love, affection, success, or even of being able to express anger counteract the effects of stressors, and to what extent do they have an independent positive effect on health?"[6] It is curious to note, however, with Miller and others, that so little work has been done on mechanisms that operate in pleasant circumstances rather than in aversive unpleasant ones. It is almost as if investigators have the idea that the normal human condition is pleasant, and stress is abnormal. What about "the chemistry of confidence," as McGuire put it, in commenting on Cousins's paper. The question deserves a better answer than I have so far seen. Being in control, free, might have been as important to that long-time editor Cousins, however unconsciously, as any laughter. As

4. Ruderman, F. A., A placebo for the doctor, *Commentary*, May 1980:54–60, 1980.
5. Cousins, N., *The healing heart*, New York: Norton, 1983.
6. Miller, N. E., Behavioral medicine: Symbiosis between laboratory and clinic, *Ann. Rev. Psychol.* 54:1–31, 1983.

Ruderman has pointed out, he was characteristically in control of his disease and his therapy.

Of course those interested in the mind will ask what really operated in Cousins's emotions. He was a man accustomed to being in control, and, as Ruderman points out, he was in charge at every point during that hospitalization: "One of the most tragic effects of major illness is the sense—the realistic sense—of loss of control over one's life, and over one's environment. . . . The seriously ill patient is deliberately rendered helpless, denied control over anything that has to do with his illness or his care."[7]

The scientific approach, which as near as I can see has not been carried out, would be to test the hypotheses clinically by controlled trials and objectively by physiological observations in a behavioral psychology laboratory. An irrational approach would be to set up clinics in movie houses or special cable TV networks specializing in the Marx Brothers, the Three Stooges, or their modern heirs! (Not Woody Allen, I think. His doubts might make some sick people worse.) But I have now seen serious discussions of the therapeutic benefit of comedians, without benefit of controlled clinical trial. Cable TV is looking for material; the health networks might alternate nutritionists, faith healers, comedians, and doctors all pitching their own therapeutic programs. To some extent I fear they already do.

It is probably useless to meditate too long on Cousins's case because it has had so much worshipful attention. His story is important because it raises questions about therapy, but no matter how enthusiastic, the dispassionate observer must find the report very little different from other reports of recovery from curses, voodoo, and other magic. Even as a report of a placebo response, it lacks validity because we know so little about the original disease. Would the *New England Journal of Medicine* have published a report of a similar outcome had it been written by a physician with as little data or by a patient less celebrated? Because so much is unknown physicians owe each other precise descriptions of such events along with all the data.

PATIENT AUTONOMY

Cousins's account raises questions about professional responsibility and the limits of patient autonomy, about how much the patient should decide. Presumably his doctors were in complete agreement with Cassell's view that the primary aim of medicine is to restore personal autonomy. I think that phrase means simply getting the patient

7. Ruderman, A placebo for the doctor.

back to where he was before he got sick, restoring the status quo. I hope it does not mean anything more, a whole repair job, so to speak. To some extent such an aim would put the physician in even more paternalistic a relationship than ever. I may want my physician to repair only my bronchi or my back and leave me a slave to my dependent neuroses. Illich has reemphasized how much medical practice and physicians have medicalized society. We may well ask whether the patient with pneumonia or an ulcer is either consciously or unconsciously asking the physician to restore his autonomy. Most sick people want to get well and, offered the choice between cimetidine and psychotherapy for a peptic ulcer, usually opt—as they should—for medicine and leave their autonomy where it was. These are matters which most physicians and patients work out as they establish a relationship. Patient autonomy must be weighed against physician authority, or responsibility.

We should not let a hard and fast rule of patient autonomy override the physician's own professional responsibility, and more important, his integrity and his beneficence. Call it paternalism if you will, but the physician is an expert, licensed by the state to apply special knowledge. It would be a lamentable abdication of responsibility if the physician did not recognize that he knows more about what is going on than the patient. While physicians have been learning to try to make the patient an equal partner in decisions about the patient's health, the equality so much talked about really does not exist in many physician-patient encounters, and we should not pretend that it does or should. A patient is a person, in Ramsey's phrase, but he is often one who is sick, upset, worried, and to some extent not the person he ordinarily is. The physician works to restore health and hopes that autonomy will follow, but he cannot always act as if patients are always rational, prudent, and equal decision-makers, particularly in an acute illness. The patient needs help, and even in a chronic illness, inequality may exist. Henderson put it well: "A patient sitting in your office, facing you, is rarely in a favorable state of mind to appreciate the precise significance of a logical statement. . . . The patient is moved by fears and by many other sentiments, and these, together with the reason, are being modified by the doctor's words and phrases, by his manner and expression."[8]

One well may ask why physicians should control the placebo. Would it not be well, for example, for a patient to give himself a placebo out of conviction? That is what Cousins did. Patient autonomy collides with professional responsibility and only after the physician has evalu-

8. Henderson, L. J., Physician and patient as a social system, *NEJM* 212:819–23, 1935.

ated the situation does patient control of placebo seem appropriate. Of course, before they go to the physician, most people will have tried home remedies, most of which are presumably placebic. Once the physician is consulted, however, his professional responsibility must play a deciding role.

A PHYSICIAN-PATIENT: FRANZ INGELFINGER

Franz Ingelfinger was editor of the *New England Journal of Medicine* in the 1960s and 1970s, and a gastroenterologist. An expert in diseases of the esophagus, to which he had devoted his life, he ironically enough developed cancer of the esophagus. All his doctors assumed that Ingelfinger knew more than they about what to do:

> Let me tell you how the lack of authoritarian decision brought agony to me and my family. About a year and a half ago it was discovered that I had an adenocarcinoma, a glandular cancer, sitting astride the gastroesophageal junction. Ironically, this had been an area of the gut to which I had paid much attention in my professional career as a clinical investigator and consultant; therefore, I can hardly imagine a more informed patient.[9]

After resection of the tumor, the question arose whether Ingelfinger should be given radiation, chemotherapy, both, or neither. Because of his knowledge in the field and because of his dominant position as editor of the premier general medical journal, his doctors asked him what he wanted them to do, and in addition many medical friends sent much contradictory advice:

> As a result, not only I but my wife, my son and daughter-in-law (both doctors), and other family members became increasingly confused and emotionally distraught. Finally, when the pangs of indecision had become nearly intolerable, one wise physician friend said, "What you need is a doctor." He was telling me to forget the information I already had and the information I was receiving from many quarters, and to seek instead a person who would dominate, who would tell me what to do, and who would in a paternalistic manner assume responsibility for my care. When that excellent advice was followed, my family and I sensed immediate and immense relief.

Ingelfinger—scientist, editor, and physician—found that he had to turn decisions over to others who would be loyal to his best inter-

9. Ingelfinger, Arrogance.

ests. The problem, of course, comes in deciding those best interests. Ingelfinger was famous, articulate, and to the end able to express what he wanted. In his own medical world he was even more powerful than Cousins, and those taking care of him had adequate reason to understand what he wanted and to know that their reputations to some extent might depend on how well he fared. (G. B. Shaw disagreed!) That is not always the case, and in the name of autonomy obscure people may suffer from misinterpretation simply because they are less able to tell what they want or their physicians are less willing to listen. Well-intentioned equality can lead to bad results if the physician does not affirm his own superior knowledge, as in the following anecdote.

A LABORER-PATIENT

In a study praising physician-patient equality, Mark Siegler tells how he let an old man die rather than force him to submit to diagnostic procedures which he did not want.[10]

Siegler tells us that the man was black and sixty-six. "Previously healthy," he had had three days of a sore throat, muscle aches, and other symptoms which suggested pneumonia to his physicians. The diagnosis was confirmed by chest X-ray, but when the patient did not respond to routine antibiotic therapy and laboratory studies suggested that an infection or a cancer might be affecting his bone marrow, further studies seemed to be in order. These were unpleasant and involved extracting some bone marrow by needle and putting a tube into the trachea to look for specific bacteria invading the respiratory tract. For reasons which were not made clear, the patient refused these diagnostic procedures, and then each of his physicians tried to persuade him to agree:

> Mr. D. became angry and agitated by this prolonged pressure, and subsequently began refusing even routine blood tests and x-rays. . . .
>
> The psychiatrist who evaluated Mr. D. concluded that although he was obviously ill and had a degree of mental impairment manifested by poor memory, he was not mentally incompetent. The psychiatrist thought that the patient understood the severity of his illness and the reasons the physicians were recommending certain tests, but that he was still making a rational choice in refusing the test.

10. Siegler, M., Clinical illness: The limits of autonomy, *Hastings Center Report* 7:12–15, 1977.

Considerable disagreement apparently ensued between Dr. Siegler and the resident physicians taking care of the patient. It was clear that "if he survived this crisis he would be able to return to a normal life and would not be an invalid or require chronic supportive care." Siegler goes on to tell how he became convinced that the patient was making a conscious rational decision to refuse a particular kind of treatment. The patient soon died, and his course was presented as a model for patient autonomy in a rather ringing fashion, or so it seems:

> The intellectual and emotional strength necessary to resist the powers of the medical system to persuade and force him to accept what they wanted to offer must have been enormous. He died a dignified death. . . . I am sadly moved that he had to expend his last measures of intellectual and physical energy in ongoing debate with his physicians.

A physician more sure of his professional responsibility might have looked at this patient in another way. He might have concluded that a sixty-six-year-old man with pneumonia who had not responded to treatment, with trouble breathing for almost a week, might not be in a state to make any rational decision if only because he might not be getting enough oxygen to his brain through his stricken lungs. Such a physician might have concluded that the patient's ability to make decisions had been so compromised that the physician had to regard the situation as an emergency. The patient had been well three days before coming to the hospital, with no story of chronic disease; I might have decided that consideration of the patient's values in such a quickly deteriorating but potentially curable disorder had little or no place. Siegler admits that had the patient been twenty-six years old instead of sixty-six, he might have acted differently: "For example, I would have demanded a more perfect 'mental status examination' and would have scrupulously checked a younger patient for evidence of a 'toxic delirium' or an acute depression. . . . I believe that I might have acted differently with a younger patient."

Siegler's discussion has rather the air of catharsis about it. He leaves at least me unable to recognize his arguments as valid: "I readily admit that my clinical judgement that the disease was rapidly progressive and almost certainly fatal further influenced me."

Siegler let the principal of radical autonomy for competent adults override clinical judgements in a way that not all will understand. The man had had an acute illness that clearly could have affected his mental ability. I conclude that the appropriate course would have been to have carried out the necessary procedures, treated the patient if at all possible, and awaited results thereafter, facing a lawsuit with equanimity. It is hard to believe that a court or jury would conclude that a man restored to health had a valid claim for damages. I certainly would have discussed the matter with the patient's wife or family, but the three-day, relatively acute course suggests that autonomy and considerations of equality should have played much less a role than they did. Aged sixty, as I write this, I hope that the now older Siegler has reevaluated the role of age in his decision-making.

What, it seems to the outside observer, was going on was that the man was afraid of pain, and instead of negotiating with the patient about his fears and concerns, the stance of patient-physician equality froze the relationship and allowed what might have been a curable disorder to lead to death.

Equality for the patient is balanced by the physician's professional integrity. His authority has to stand for something. A Catholic physician will not be asked to carry out an abortion, and patient equality meets its limit in what the physician as person and as professional can accept as reasonable.

Moreover the patient is not and cannot be an equal partner. He has an overriding interest, greater than that of the doctor, in getting well. The old adage has it that the doctor who treats himself has a fool for a patient and a fool for a physician. If that is true, as I believe it is, the patient is less likely to make adequate choices unless guided by his physician. Ingelfinger and Cousins show us different sides of this problem. We should continue to tell such stories and to ponder them.

BENEFICENCE

Thomasma offers one way out in his attempt to balance the shortcomings of the patient autonomy ideal and the medical paternalistic habit.[11] He emphasizes the importance of beneficence, acting for the benefit of another and responding to a plea for help. He also takes into account the values of the physician who must make choices in the care of his patient. In a sense, clothed with different elements and lacking any imposition of values or decisions made "in the best interests of patients without their participation" both physician and patient respect their own values. Thomasma reawakens the notion of the importance of "moral character" in educating physicians. I confess to believing that the physician must do more than be a passive guide. He has the expertise and training to help the patient choose the best way, as the patient sees it.

11. Thomasma, D. C., Beyond medical paternalism and patient autonomy: A model of physician conscience for the physician-patient relationship, *Ann. Intern. Med.* 98:243–48, 1983; and Limitations of the autonomy model for the doctor-patient relationship, *Pharos* 46:2–5, 1983.

9

Objections to
the Placebo

Objections to placebo come on grounds which a non-philosopher might tautologically call ethical, economic and consequential. The first is concerned mainly with the nature of the act, with lying and truth-telling, in philosophical terms a deontological objection. The other two objections are more utilitarian. Should people spend money on "useless" drugs? What are the consequences of the physician's believing in, and the patient's trusting in, a pill?

On the whole most ethicists disapprove of placebos, but physicians writing about the matter usually approve of them at least when placebos are used selectively, to benefit the patient. It is the old tension between theory and practice. The term *ethicist* has come into view over the past decade, and refers to someone, usually a philosopher, who is able to decide what is "right" and what is "wrong," or, to remain charitable, "better" and "worse." In medicine today it is usually applied to someone other than a physician who judges or at least evaluates how doctors act with patients, but who himself does not take care of patients. The term parallels *physicist* and is supposed to convey the same relation to ethics that the scientist has to physics.

TRUTH-TELLING AND LYING

Most ethical objections to the placebo come on the basis of truth-telling. Truth-telling has been a classical and recently recurrent theme in biomedical ethics, but it has been dominated by consideration of the dying patient. Discussions at the extreme are likely to give too stark and even a misleading view, full as they are of the contrast between the helpless dying patient dominated by his paternalistic physician who withholds facts to control the truth. The sharp light cast by

117

the question, "Should dying patients be told the truth?" bleaches out any chiaroscuro of the placebo picture.

The Dying Patient

For a long time well-meaning physicians felt that it was their duty to shield their patients from harm, particularly from the agonizing depression that they felt would follow news of impending death. Davidoff, a noted neurosurgeon, was typical.

If the patient has a very malignant tumor, I tell the relatives that a tumor was found and removed, and that the patient has withstood the procedure well. Mostly, the relatives will then immediately ask,
"Was it malignant, Doctor?" My answer is, "that it was a growth within the brain substance itself, and that the separation of brain tissue from tumor was not too clearly defined; . . . that, however, the final judgment as to prognosis cannot be made until after a report by the laboratory which may take 4 or 5 days." When the laboratory report arrives and perchance bears out the most optimistic interpretation of the gross findings, this can be transmitted joyously to the family and even to the patient. If the growth proves to be really malignant, some responsible member of the family must be told. Whether the patient is told or not will then depend on what he wants to know. The questions and answers may be something like this:
Patient: "Well, Doctor, how did it go?"
Doctor: "Fine, fine, everything went very well."
Patient: "Was everything removed that doesn't belong there?"
Doctor: "Yes, it's all out."[1]

Medical practice changes slowly, and over the four decades since that passage was written, most physicians have come to agree that dying patients, or patients with cancer or other potentially fatal illnesses, should be told the truth. A vast literature has grown up around this tenet, and Richard Cabot has been enshrined as its American saint.

Richard Cabot

A formidable clinician and teacher, Richard Cabot was careful to emphasize that a true or false impression can be conveyed without words.

Now, I was brought up, as I suppose every physician is, to use what are called placebos, that is bread pills, subcutaneous injections of a few drops of water (supposed by the patient to be morphine), and

1. Davidoff, L., What one neurosurgeon does. In *Should the patient know the truth?* New York: Springer, 1955, pp. 88–92.

other devices for acting upon a patient's symptoms through his
mind. . . . It never occurred to me until I had given a great many
"placebos" that, if they are to be really effective, they must deceive
the patient. . . . If the patient knows what we are up to when we
give him a bread pill it will have no effect on him. If he is dyspeptic
he must believe that we consider the medicine we give likely to act
upon his stomach and not merely upon his stomach through his
mind. Otherwise it will do him no good. Suppose we said to him: "I
give you this pill for its mental effect. It has no action on the stomach;" would he be likely to get benefit from it? No, it is only when
through the placebo one deceives the patient that any effect is produced. It is only when we act like quacks that our placebos work.[2]

Richard Cabot's comments have been widely read. He argues appropriately, and many others have followed him, that the patient who
gets a pill will learn to expect a pill for other complaints, that physicians thereby perpetuate false ideas about disease and its cure.

To back this idea up Cabot tells the story of

An unfortunate patient was floating around from one clinic to another, as happens now and then when diagnosis and treatment are
unsuccessful. This poor woman complained that she had a lizard in
her stomach, that she felt his movements distinctly, and that they
rendered her life unbearable. Doctor after doctor had assured her
that the thing was impossible, that no such animal could subsist in-
side a human being, that the trouble was wholly a fanciful one, and
that she must do her best to think of it no more. But all such explanations and reassurances were of no avail.

Cabot tells how suggestion did not work, how a friend of his had
told her that she indeed had a lizard in her stomach and that he could
give her a chemical which would dissolve the lizard "and allow the resulting substance to be excreted by the kidney." What in fact the physician gave the woman was methylene blue, a dye which is absorbed
from the intestine and then filtered by the kidneys to give a deep blue
color to the urine: "The woman took the medicine and perceived to
her amazement and delight that a blue color was imparted to her
urine, recognized that the lizard must have been dissolved, and was at
once free from all her symptoms."

Cabot then goes on to tell how symptoms recurred, "another lizard
grew," and the patient

turned up at still another Out-Patient clinic under the charge of a
very honest physician, to whom she told her story. . . . The doctor

2. Cabot, R. C., The use of truth and falsehood in medicine, (as edited by Katz, J.)
Conn. Med. 42:189–94, 1978.

went one step further than anyone had gone before; he investigated not only what was not the matter with her, but what the trouble actually was. He found that she had an excess of gastric juice in her stomach, the irritation of which gave the gnawing and scratching feeling which she attributed to the presence of a lizard. Having discovered this fact he proceeded to treat her for this trouble, which he succeeded in curing, and after that time the lizard never grew again.

I assume that Richard Cabot was the "very honest physician" in his tale. I do not know how long his follow-up lasted. I do know that measurements of gastric acid have never proven of much diagnostic value. I also know that at his time measurements of gastric acid were too primitive to mean much. Indeed in the 1980s, despite much more precise gastric acid measurements, gastroenterologists have given up any belief that the amount of acid in the stomach is ordinarily of any diagnostic significance. I therefore suspect that Cabot substituted one form of belief, this time in a measurement, for another. I imagine that the woman's cure was short-lived, but the confrontation between the woman's belief system, which we might well suppose was European peasant in origin, and that of the rational, truthful, scientific Bostonian physician of the twentieth century is wonderful to contemplate. It is not that different from the confrontation of Beaumont, another New Englander, with Alexis St. Martin, a French-Canadian voyageur. As a gastroenterologist I am gratified to see that both Cabot and Beaumont turned to the stomach. Beaumont imposed his search for facts and "the truth" on St. Martin by studying his gastric acid over and over again and, even in the last stages of their relationship, pursuing him over great distances to convince him to undergo more studies of his stomach. To help his patient Richard Cabot studied her gastric secretion to convince her that the acid was the source of her trouble. Beaumont was among the first to show that acid was present in the stomach; Cabot, like many of his time, used gastric analysis diagnostically and in a sense therapeutically. At any rate I believe that Cabot relieved his patient, at least temporarily, by imposing his own system of beliefs with its own therapy. (In Chapter 10, I discuss the role of "lizards" in folk medicine, to suggest that Cabot's patient was not as bizarre as modern physicians might think.)

Cabot comes down against placebos and for telling the truth in all circumstances. He has had great influence, but he may have had a personal reason for justifying truth-telling in all circumstances.

Cabot and his brothers. Richard Cabot is a man whose writings I have much admired since my medical school days. His book, *The Art of Min-*

istering to the Sick,[3] written with Russell Dicks, chaplain at the Massachusetts General Hospital, has some remarkable insights which have been a guide to me for almost forty years and which I reread from time to time, though I do not share their eschatological viewpoint. I have recommended the book over and over again to Yale medical students. Cabot's strictures on lying, however, I find less congenial, not because I favor mendacity, but because they seem somewhat self-righteous, even sanctimonious. I knew nothing about Richard Cabot as a person, except that he was the founder of the "CPCs," educational exercises, clinico-pathological cases, correlating what the doctor discussing a case thinks was wrong with the patient during life, with what the pathologist has found after the patient had died. They have long been a highlight of the *New England Journal of Medicine*.

It was with astonishment then that while I was writing this book I read an article in the *Harvard Medical Alumni Bulletin* by Patricia Ward about Richard and his brother Hugh.[4] Both were graduates of Harvard College and its medical school. Hugh went on to become professor of surgery at the University of Michigan. A urologist with a skeptical and humorous view of medicine, he is quoted as saying, "There are fools, damn fools, and then there is my brother, Richard." And Ward tells us, "Richard's positive nature and absolute certainty of being right made him an ideal teacher."

He must have had a lot of common sense. About high blood pressure he wrote, "Those who are subject to unavoidable financial or domestic worries and those who have to earn their living by muscular work usually succumb within a year or two."

But Richard Cabot was not always as right as his subsequent canonization might suggest. In 1910 he sponsored a program of catharsis for the treatment of drug addiction, characterized by others as "diarrhea, delirium, and damnation." Of more interest, Ms. Ward tells us that Richard believed in celibacy and "stoutly denied that anyone needed to know more about sex." He "steadfastly rejected any suggestion that the sex instinct was basic to human nature." His marriage was confessedly and proudly celibate.

More important, in relation to his insistence on always telling the truth, is the story of another brother Ted, who, in the days before insulin, was slowly and apparently painfully dying of diabetes.

Ward puts it this way:

> On one of Richard's visits in late October, when Ted had experienced a bout of fever his physicians could not explain, Ted, his

---

3. Cabot, R. C., and Dicks, R. L., *The art of ministering to the sick*, New York: MacMillan, 1947.

4. Ward, P. S., The medical brothers Cabot: Of truth and consequence, *Harvard Med.* 56:30–39, 1982.

parents, and Richard agreed that Richard should act to end his suffering. Several days before the appointed time, Ted said a goodbye to his mother which she described as "enough to live on and live by for the rest of her life." He struck a note in this farewell, she said, "That brings all life and death itself into perfect harmony and to be with him is to be with God."

Ted was thirty-two, Richard only twenty-five when they made the awesome decision that Ted should die on November 10, 1893. How much of Richard Cabot's insistence on truth-telling and absolute frankness had to do with justifying for the rest of his life the decision to kill his brother? Was his insistence on telling the truth to the dying a life-long attempt to make his act a model for others? We can only conjecture in the absence of journals. Surely putting his brother to death must have lived with Cabot and influenced what he thought and wrote about these matters.

Could Hans Zinsser, a contemporary of Cabot, have been referring to Cabot when he wrote that "a well-known American physician who was at the same time—to my mind—a canting moralist held on occasion that absolute, uncompromising truthfulness is the only justifiable position, however cruel."[5] He added: "The truth can be exaggerated when the doctor talks to a hopeless patient. . . . One must pick one's situations and one's cases, and adjust the truth to the judgement of wise kindness."

I do not want to diminish the message by attacking the writer. Many of us generalize from our own experience and consciously and unconsciously justify our acts and lives, offering rules from what we prefer. Cabot's story is a perplexing one to me and worth pondering. At any rate, telling the truth to every patient, and especially bringing the bad news to the dying, has become a value that is no longer publically questioned. Truth-telling has become a greater virtue than mercy, although some experienced physicians still try to weigh the feather of benevolence and beneficence against this harder virtue.

What Is Truth in Medical Practice?

It would be a brave physician who tried to answer this question, but he does have an obligation to transmit his specialized knowledge to his patients as he understands it. As Bonhoeffer put it, "'Telling the truth' means something different according to the particular situation in which one stands. Account must be taken of one's relationship at each particular time . . . in each case the truth which this speech conveys is also different."[6]

5. Zinsser, H., *As I remember him: The biography of R. S.*, Boston: Little Brown, 1941, pp. 140–41.
6. Bonhoeffer, D., *Ethics*, ed. E. Bethge, New York: Macmillan, 1962, p. 326.

For the physician, that is transmitting the medical facts as he knows them, however difficult it may be to agree on those facts. Bok gives us a practical, useful guide: "The moral question of whether you are lying or not is not settled by establishing the truth or falsity of what you say. In order to *settle* this question, we must know whether you *intend your statement to mislead*."[7] That emphasis on intent sets a boundary to pertinent discussion. There are many kinds of lies, from the practices of Davidoff to the current emphasis on "truth-telling."

Three definitions of truth are given: (1) correspondence with facts; (2) internal consistency or coherence with other judgments that are believed to be true; or (I think best) (3) a pragmatic test of their utility. I will settle on intent, given the difficulty in understanding facts. Even if I recognize the strength of Marilyn Smith's argument that since one's intentions are strictly private, the person lied to will never know the intent. "If I force you to answer whether you are intending to mislead or not, what is to prevent you from further intending to deceive, that is, from lying."[8]

Lies and Lies

Medical practice has moved far from the views of physicians like Leo Davidoff who kept knowledge of their cancer from patients who were soon to die, simply to give them peace of mind. Keeping the diagnosis from a dying patient, however, is not quite the same as giving him a placebo to relieve his pain. The proverbial prudent man would choose to know that he is dying; he might regard as a trivial professional consideration whether an ulcer that brought him to his doctor was duodenal or gastric in location. He might not care to learn all the differences between them and that a gastric ulcer runs a minuscule chance of being a cancer. The person who comes to a physician for pain in his belly might well be as satisfied with immediate relief as with the slow acquisition of arcane medical knowledge. After being relieved, he might choose to know more.

The dying person, nowadays always a "patient," needs to know what his doctor knows to make final plans, and is usually harmed by not knowing his outlook. The anxiety which may come, the grief or depression or rage, or other feelings are potential problems which, it has been argued, are less important than those which arise when the benevolent physician tries to prevent anxiety by hiding the approach of death. That is really quite a different matter from trying to bring relief to the patient in pain. With a placebo such a patient has the likelihood of benefit, of pain relief, even if he is deprived of myriad scien-

7. Bok, S., *Lying: Moral choice in public and private life*, New York: Pantheon, 1978, p. 6.
    8. Smith, M., The white lie, unpublished.

tific details and the whole truth. The context of truth-telling in these circumstances is quite different from that in the dying patient, if only because the situation is not, after all, an irrevocable one.

There are lies and lies. Even the firmest ethicists will agree that some deceptions are trivial, such as praising a tie or dress, a lecture or a role in a play. They keep the social machinery oiled, and do little harm. Other lies, of course, are major, and it is on these that most commentators seize. In looking at medical practice, common sense should help us separate the trivial from the important. Reassuring a patient in acute pain who must undergo an emergency operation that everything will be all right hardly falls into the same category as telling a patient with a gastric cancer that he has a little ulcer.

The "hairy hand": Is reassurance a guarantee? In a famous contract law case, *Hawkins* v. *McGee*, read by all law students and known irreverently as the "hairy hand" case, a suit concerned how much of a guarantee—or in legal terms, a warranty—Dr. McGee, a surgeon, had made for the success of his operation.[9]

A young man had had a scarred right hand from a burn for which McGee took a graft from his chest wall. Complications led to a postoperative course which was long and troublesome rather than the easy time that had been expected.

Before the operation the plaintiff claimed that he and his father went to the defendant's office and that the surgeon, when asked how long the boy would be in the hospital, answered, "Three or four days, not over four; then the boy can go home and it will be just a few days when he will go back to work with a good hand."

The questions that the courts and lawyers have looked at many times since then have been whether McGee had really promised something or whether he was simply offering reassurance. Usually, but not always, it has been agreed that doctors do not warranty their services and such statements as those of Dr. McGee's are simply good-hearted reassurance. The courts have usually held that the uncertainties of medical practice make it impossible for a physician-patient agreement to be like a commercial contract. The physician cannot insure his patient's good health or satisfaction and should not be held liable for what is in essence simple human reassurance. The rare times when the courts have upheld a suit for a "contract to cure" have involved an egregious and self-seeking claim on the part of the physician about what he could do for the patient.

9. *Hawkins* v. *McGee*, Supreme Court of New Hampshire, 1929, cited in *Contracts*, ed. J. R. Dawson, W. B. Harvey, and S. D. Henderson, Mineola, N.Y.: Foundation Press, 1982, pp. 1–4.

Truth-telling and comforting. Grimly holding on to truth-telling as the most important ethic, many observers fail to permit what seem to some practitioners to be common-sense decisions. At present most philosophical commentators give telling the truth a higher priority than relieving pain. But I sometimes think that, to use their terms, "goods" may be more important than "rights" to the patient in pain; the patient may prefer relief to "the truth."

There is much to be said on these matters, but I emphasize that patients are all different: some can tolerate all the truth particularly if it is couched in hopeful terms. For many denial and suppression prevent the honest dialogue between physician and patient that is our goal. For others denial is a useful merciful reaction. Not everyone can handle the unvarnished truth. Cousins asks, "Is it possible to communicate negative information in such a way that it is received by the patient as a challenge rather than as a death sentence?"[10]

Liberty may have its limits, and the current valuation which puts autonomy ahead of health may not last forever. Is the patient in chronic pain the same person that he was in good health? The patient with cancer, kept alive by hyperalimentation for months, dependent on others in the hospital, turned from side to side to prevent bed sores, may be "infantilized." He may not be able to make absolutely rational decisions, or decisions that he might have made three or four months before when he was still in good health. We have to respect his decisions even in that helpless state, asking permission, talking to him, and discussing matters of mutual concern. But we have to remember the enormous capacity of people to adapt to almost any circumstances. The patient long in the hospital who has undergone several operations, who has been fed by tubes in vein and gullet, and who can no longer speak because of the tubes or who is confused by his long stay, is not in the same state as when he was in good health. Can we physicians really assess his decisions when all he can do is nod his head or grimace? Are those decisions the same he would have made when he was well? That is why living wills or the "durable power of attorney" have come into vogue. They insure that someone else we trust to be loyal to our best interests as we see them when we are in our full power will help to make decisions about us if we are unconscious, deranged, or just childlike and helpless.

Physicians try to restore their patients to health, to bring them back to a state where they can make free decisions. After all, if autonomy has been narrowed by disease, if the patient in pain is not the same person as the patient without pain, (something physicians know from daily experience), then enhancing autonomy without relieving pain

10. Cousins, N., *The Healing Heart*, New York: Norton, 1983, p. 135.

may not provide the greatest benefit. Physicians are hardened by day-to-day demands of patients who talk not of long-term goals but of feeling better, and who seem ready to trade freedom for relief. They hear over and over again, "You are the doctor. You decide." They take that acquiescence to be the universal condition of the sick, not the claimed autonomy that they read about. Physicians usually agree on professional beneficence because they find that their patients do not want to think quite so much about these matters as philosophers claim.

I emphasize that I believe that physicians should always aim at telling the truth, and that often means saying to someone, "You are dying." That often means for the physician confronting the truth himself, that his patient is dying, and that he should not do everything to prolong that dying. As I write this, I am fresh from a stint taking care of patients on our hospital wards, and I have been reminded of how the inability to confront the fact that the patient is dying leads to great torment, for patient and family, and to uneasiness for the physician.

On the wards of our hospitals in the mid–1980s lie a number of patients with AIDS, in the prolonged throes of their death agony. That may sound like an exaggeration. One has only to see a thirty-year-old man—jaundiced, with diarrhea he cannot control, breathing (gasping rather) with the benefit of oxygen, sustained by tubes into his heart to keep him alive, semiconscious if not disoriented, abandoned by friends and visited by medical personnel garbed in yellow robes and masked in white with gloved hands—to wonder whether a frank admission on the part of the physician that there is no turning back, that the patient is dying, would not be wiser—and more merciful. Certainly the insistence on doing everything possible, even when we know that no miracle is even in sight, seems cruel.

Autonomy and the Placebo

Thomasma suggests that patient autonomy had its origins in the civil rights movement of the 1960s.[11] The patient autonomy movement may wrongfully have carried over into the medical relationship adversarial preconceptions in tone, which imply that the physician is trying to put something over on the patient. The adversary relationship surely is no model for physician-patient care, nor has it ever been. Indeed it is adopting an adversary relationship that sometimes provokes physicians into using the placebo as a challenge. That is just the opposite of how the benevolent placebo should be used.

Illness or disease weakens the patient's control over his own body.

11. Thomasma, D., Beyond medical paternalism and patient autonomy, *Ann. Intern. Med.* 98:243–48, 1983.

Newton sees such loss of control as an increased effect of gravity in the presence of disease: "The body, usually transparent, suddenly becomes opaque. It takes on weight; where before the arm was weightless, reaching for the book it now is heavy."[12] The first control that the physician must restore to the patient is control over his own body, and I would add that only later should we worry about the more abstract notions of choice and informed consent. To some extent, when we talk about control and autonomy, we must be sure we are talking about the same thing.

Paternalism, Strong and Weak

Arguments against the placebo as a lie often bring up the question of paternalism, something of which physicians used to feel proud and for which now they are usually attacked. Paternalism may be defined as an action taken by one person in what he takes to be the best interest of another without the explicit consent of the person to be benefitted. It comes in two forms, at least for physicians: (1) *Strong* paternalism is an action taken *against* the expressed wishes of a patient, to save his life, for example. A classic example is the young man burned beyond hope of ever being active again, who wanted to die and who said so, but whose life was saved against his will. (2) *Weak* paternalism, Thomasma tells us, is an action taken by a physician in the best interest of a patient on the basis of what the physician presumes the patient would want if asked or—more defensively—choosing for patients whose mental status precludes their being asked. Keeping a comatose patient alive is the usual example.[13]

We should distinguish between *not* telling a patient about theories one may have about how a placebo works from more major kinds of paternalism. Again, to repeat, there seems quite a difference between holding to oneself a theory that placebos may work because faith in them generates endorphins and not telling a patient that he has cancer. Still, if we assume that the patient with pain wants first to lose his pain, his self-interest might dictate our saying, "I don't know how this pill works, but I would like you to take it anyway because I believe that it will help you," rather than exploring all possible avenues. It might be argued that rational persons would choose to lose their pain even at the cost of not knowing everything, at the loss of free choice, rather than to continue to suffer and run the risk of diagnostic tests.

Allen Buchanan brings fresh arguments against medical paternalism.[14] He argues persuasively that withholding information about

12. Newton, L., The healing of the person, *Conn. Med.* 41:641–46, 1977.
13. Thomasma, Beyond medical paternalism.
14. Buchanan, A., Medical paternalism, *J. Philos. Pub. Affairs* 7:370–90, 1978.

cancer, for example, for the patient's benefit has only a shallow foundation: (1) the judgment that telling the truth would result in depression or guilt is a psychiatric generalization made for individual patients by physicians not trained as psychiatrists; (2) it is doubtful that even psychiatrists have the skills or information to make such predictions; and (3) the paternalistic physician assumes that suicide, if that is the outcome of knowing the truth, is not a rational choice for the terminally ill.

Buchanan further argues that withholding information from the parents of a defective newborn in order to spare them the misery or guilt of making a decision to let that newborn die (1) suggests that physician makes the parents into patients as much as the child; and (2) assumes that it is the duty of the physician to minimize or to prevent harm to the family as well as to the patient. Physicians have not taken on the obligation of treating the relatives, Buchanan reminds us, and the relatives may not choose to be patients. Once we recognize that the physician really has no claim to such a wide-ranging role, the absurdity of such apparently altruistic decisions becomes clear. The physician who would make such a decision must claim to know a great deal about the parents, the other children, and be able to arrive at a justifiable prediction of harm. The physician is capable, as Buchanan emphasizes, of judging what will harm or benefit a patient on the strictly technical level, but he has no more right than anyone else to make judgments about another human being's moral or spiritual life.

Turning to the distinctions between ordinary and extraordinary measures, he points out that the judgments called upon are purely technical, the feasibility or the utility of one machine over another, for example. Making the distinctions among extraordinary measures on a technical basis obscures the fact that decisions are being made. Buchanan cautions that such moral decisions should not be made simply and solely by physicians hiding under the guise of feasibility. I find his arguments persuasive as far as the major issues are concerned. He does not comment on the placebo, but he provides a rich background for our thinking.

Altruistic Deception

White lies. Bok puts placebos in the category of "white lies," common, trivial and benevolent in that they are not meant to injure and are of little moral import.[15] Placebos, she says, are advocated as bringing "a more substantial benefit or avoiding a real harm." In none of her writings on lying does she condemn the placebo as such; instead she argues mainly from the consequences of their being given.

15. Bok, *Lying.*

She suggests, for example, that giving placebos will enhance people's dependence on pills and drugs. She fears that the patient who finds out that he has been deceived will lose confidence in both physicians and bonafide medicines. I do not know whether she is saying that patients will then not take pills that they need or that their lack of faith will make the pill less effective.

Bok's arguments rest on utilitarian premises. Arguing from the consequences for *other* patients is not the same as saying that the placebo is harmful for the patient who receives it. Physicians have not yet been asked to make such a utilitarian calculus on the social harm outweighing the individual benefit. (To some extent, of course, that is exactly what is beginning to happen in the era of diagnostic related groups. These require the physician to look at the social harm which will come from spending money on too many tests and ask him to examine whether the benefit to the hospital of not doing tests and so saving money is greater than the benefit to the patient, however small, of carrying out more diagnostic steps.)

Bok also argues that acceptance of a placebo can "encourage other kinds of deception in medicine" for benevolent reasons. She agrees that telling a patient "I believe these pills may help you" is not a lie or deceitful in itself. Indeed the physician who knows, or expects, that the placebo will relieve pain as well as anything else is not "lying" or deceiving the patient as to his own frame of mind. But Bok regards the setting of the doctor's office or hospital, the clinical context of the physician-patient meeting, as "deceptive even if the words are so general as not to be lies."

I am not sure what "the setting" says except about the decorating taste of the physician. The general atmosphere is meant to be one of help, and that is what the placebo is all about. She argues that information that is material and important is withheld, such as the fact that the physician does not know what the patient's problem is when he gives a placebo. As a nonphysician, Bok may be too much of a diagnostic activist, with too much faith in what doctors can do, even with current diagnostic and therapeutic apparatus.

The physician need not know, indeed it may be in everyone's interest for him *not* to try to know, what is going on beyond a general assessment that it is nothing serious. Some ethicists have argued, on the other hand, that not to tell the patient that his faith may stimulate endorphins is still to deceive the patient. The consequences of such an approach can only be imagined. We will be back in the era of faith healing. But it will put the onus for getting better back on the patient, which is apparently what the patient-equality and people's medicine are all about. Bok goes no further than to call such an approach undesirable. Warning that no outright lie should ever be told, she does not put a placebo in the same category as deceiving patients about a serious illness or about their outlook.

Philosophers' Conclusion

Bok seems reluctant to leave room for the placebo, with some limitations under the category of "altruistic deception." She reminds us that Plato permitted lies to the sick and dying as examples of benevolent deception. Bok concludes:

> 1) Placebo should be used only after a careful diagnosis; 2) no active placebo should be used, merely inert ones; 3) no outright lie should be told and questions should be answered honestly; 4) placebo should never be given to patients who have asked not to receive them; 5) placebo should never be used when treatment is clearly called for or all possible alternatives have not been weighed.

Brody has written a definitive book on placebo, but even though he is both a philosopher and a physician, he leaves me uncertain of his stance.[16] In a later paper he accepts the similarity between a physician deceiving his patient with a placebo and the magician deceiving an audience with his illusions.[17] This analogy to a magician is used by a number of writers, but I do not accept it as a useful or accurate metaphor. The intent of the physician giving a placebo is to relieve pain or suffering; that of the magician is to deceive, for pleasure. The analogy transmits information which is not helpful to an understanding of the placebo and misinterprets the intent of the physician or what should be his intent. The audience pays to be deceived for its pleasure, but the patient comes to the physician for relief. We come back to the same question, of course, whether the primary intent of the patient runs along the lines of "First, tell me the truth" or "First, make me feel better."

Brody comes down in favor of the nondeceptive use of the placebo and offers a useful comment: "Healing comes not from the lie itself, but rather from the relationship between healer and patient, and the latter's own capacity for self-healing via symbolic and psychological approaches as via biological intervention."

Simmons, on the other hand, wholly disapproves of placebos from the legal and ethical standpoint, and from the consequences that flow from them.

> Placebo use necessitates deceptive practices which obscure the truth. . . . No therapy should be administered to a patient deliber-

---

16. Brody, H., *Placebos and the philosophy of medicine,* Chicago: University of Chicago Press, 1980.

17. Brody, H., The lie that heals, *Ann. Intern. Med.* 97:112–18, 1982.

ately to achieve a placebo effect unless they know the nature of both their "disease" and the "remedy." . . . The physician ought to make it clear that there is no chemical reason why the placebo might work, but the studies have shown that inert substances might psychologically benefit the patient. . . . In other words, where the patient agrees to therapy *understanding* that the physiological benefit might be triggered by a psychological response, there is no deception.[18]

She leaves little room for the placebo, it seems to me. She asks a great deal from the patient, however, more than many want.

Byerly, a philosopher and not a physician recognizes the dilemma of trying to exploit the placebo effect which depends "essentially on deception, on a subject's having false beliefs."[19] To define the false belief is the problem. The physician says, "The pill should help you, but I don't know how" and the patient believes what he says. Byerly does not resolve the ethical issue, concluding that "perhaps placebos are best exploited in cases of doubt." His example is something like vitamin C in preventing the common cold, possibly helpful and without obvious harm. Using the least dangerous of a choice of drugs as a placebo, for Byerly, seems reasonable at least by implication, but he does not record a strong opinion.

Physicians' Conclusions

Most physicians of an earlier time agreed in having no problem with the benevolent deception of the placebo because of their clinical experience.

Henderson, a Harvard Medical School scientist, spoke for them:

A patient sitting in your office, facing you, is rarely in a favorable state of mind to appreciate the precise significance of a logical statement. . . . The patient is moved by fears and by many other sentiments, and these, together with reason, are being modified by the doctor's words and phrases, by his manner and expression. . . . The physician should see to it that the patient's sentiments do not act upon his sentiments and, above all, do not thereby modify his behavior, and he should endeavor to act upon the patient's sentiments according to a well-considered plan. . . . When you talk with a patient you should listen, first, for what he wants to tell; secondly, for what he does not want to tell; thirdly, for what he cannot tell . . . . The patient will eagerly scrutinize and rationalize what you

18. Simmons, B., Problems in deceptive medical procedures: An ethical and legal analysis of the administration of placebos, *J. Med. Ethics* 4:172–81, 1978.

19. Byerly, H., Explaining and exploiting placebo effects, *Persp. Biol. Med.* 19:423-36, 1976.

say, that he will carry it away with him, that he will turn your phrases over and over in his mind, seeking persistently for shades of meaning that you never thought of. . . . Above all, remember that it is meaningless to speak of telling the truth, the whole truth, nothing but the truth to a patient. . . . If you recognize the duty of telling the truth to the patient, you range yourself outside the class of biologist, with lawyers and philosophers. The idea that the truth, the whole truth, and nothing but the truth can be conveyed to the patient is an example of false abstraction, of that fallacy called by Whitehead, "the fallacy of misplaced concreteness."[20]

It is not a matter of the physician saying that he can make judgments no one else can make, but a matter of dealing with the real world, and real patients. The most thoughtful physicians have used the placebo as much for its symbolic value as for any attempt to deceive.

For example, Leslie in 1954 wrote, "In our discussion we have attempted first to establish that the use of the placebo entails the use of deception, then that this deception is permissible since it is for the benefit of the patient."[21] In 1982 Leslie added, "Deception is as integral to the placebo as copper is to bronze. Should we not accept the pragmatic view and in good conscience continue the judicious use of the invaluable placebo?"[22]

Silber, another physician, divides placebo use into two groups, those that "build-down" and those that "build-up."[23] Presumably the first is in confrontation, in the adversarial mode, telling a patient, "You have nothing wrong with you if a placebo helps you," whereas the second is given in the beneficent mode as a gift. He approves of placebo therapy as a form of communication "that says something that words cannot say at one particular moment. In the nature of this phenomenon, I see a justification for placebo therapy."

Adler and Hammett agree with the majority view that a lie keeps the patient ignorant of all relevant factors and therefore keeps him from self-determination.[24] Keeping the diagnosis of cancer and therefore the probability of an early death from a patient is no longer acceptable to these writers or, I suspect, to very many modern physi-

20. Henderson, L. J., Physician and patient as a social system, *NEJM* 212:819–23, 1935.

21. Leslie, A., Ethics and practice of placebo therapy, *Amer. J. Med.* 16:854–62, 1954.

22. Leslie, A., Letter, *Ann. Intern. Med.* 97:781, 1982.

23. Silber, T. J., Placebo therapy: The ethical dimension, *JAMA* 242:245–46, 1979.

24. Adler, H. M., and Hammett, V. O., The doctor-patient relationship revisited: Analysis of the placebo effect, *Ann. Intern. Med.* 78:595–98, 1973.

cians. We injure the patient whom we so deceive. We deprive him of the chance to dispose of his possessions or his remaining time in ways that, knowing the truth, he might have chosen. But Adler and Hammett implicitly approve of the placebo as helping to form a "group system" and improving the doctor-patient relationship, matters which I will discuss later.

Phillips, a professor of family practice, offers a typical medical assessment.

> It is the net effect of the health and hope the physician can offer the patient that justifies the special relationship between the two. Nothing but the truth would prove a miserable medicine. . . .
>
> What deception that is necessary for the prescription of a placebo cannot be judged right or wrong without a situation assessment of the desired outcomes.[25]

Physicians and ethicists should continue to talk, but they probably will never completely agree about the ethics of giving placebos. Presumably no ethicist will disagree with Simmons's objections, but no practicing physician will be completely comfortable with a stand so uncompromising. Physicians rarely understand how many drugs that they use everyday work. The patient—or physician—who demands to know how each drug works would deny himself the benefits of aspirin, morphine, or placebo. The physician who emphasizes the individual relationship and "the intelligent and sensitive management of each clinical situation" will use placebos, however much ethicists will argue with that approach.

For Lipkin, another practicing physician who has thought much about such matters, "The real problem is that ethicists deal with generalizations about problems and fail to take into account that it is always dangerous to apply a generalization to a particular situation. The moment of truth for the doctor is when face-to-face with a person in trouble. To generalize about individuals and prescribe identically is obvious nonsense."[26]

This point, that the physician learns to deal generally with disease first and then to apply the different remedies for different persons, is something that ethicists working in a vacuum do not readily perceive. In that sense giving placebos, like shading the truth, needs to be considered in relation to individuals rather than as generalizations. Not everyone has plans and projects to complete. Many people seem to live from day to day. In the long philosophical tradition ethicists

25. Phillips, W. R., Patients, pills, and professionals: The ethics of placebo therapy, *Pharos* 21–25, 1981.

26. Lipkin, M., letter, June 6, 1984.

sometimes regard the man on the bus as very much like the philosophers themselves.

Leslie suggests that placebos may be used (1) to wean patients off
narcotics, (2) to manage the terminally ill, (3) to substitute for drugs
which may confuse the picture, and (4) to make a temporary concession to patients.[27] Silber is more concerned with the physician's motives and suggests that a placebo may be used (1) as an act of communication as part of the total patient-physician relationship and (2) as
part of a plan to move the patient toward better health.[28]

Katz, certainly as impassioned a believer in truth-telling as there is,
asks the question in another, more helpful way:

> Should placebos be left to faith-healers and should physicians in-
> stead swear allegiance to new gods of science? Put another way,
> should physicians extend their assistance to all "suffering" human-
> ity or only to that group which they can treat with their scientific
> knowledge? . . .
>
> If placebos have a place in the practice of medicine, the physi-
> cians must appreciate more fully that placebos are not innocuous,
> that they can do much harm; for example, by becoming a means
> for hurriedly doing something in order to see the next patient,
> when nothing, except careful explanation need be provided; by
> not allowing the healing power of nature to take its course and
> instead prescribing active "placebos" which can produce iatro-
> genic ailments that require further treatment; by making persons
> through placebo treatments dependent on physicians, confirming
> them in the status of patients when instead their "recovery" could
> have been accomplished through reliance on the person's own re-
> cuperative powers; by blinding physicians to recommend with en-
> thusiasm remedies of no value, and disregarding in the process less
> detrimental alternatives.[29]

Katz recognizes how too great restriction on the use of a placebo may
interfere with cure.

ECONOMIC OBJECTIONS

The economic argument is often used against giving a placebo. Patients who take "useless medicines" will be put to needless expense in
paying for "inactive" drugs. Bok suggests correctly that millions of

27. Leslie, Letter.
28. Silber, Placebo therapy.
29. Katz, J., *The silent world of the doctor and patient,* New York: Free Press, 1984.

dollars are spent on placebos and placebic medicines. I add that many procedures as well as medicines are given as reassurance rather than as placebo. The thought is not that "this procedure or this diagnostic investigation will relieve the patient's distress," but rather that "the results of the procedure will surely prove negative and when I tell the patient that the test is normal, his anxiety will be relieved, and that in turn will diminish his pain." It is important to recognize that the procedure carried out to reassure both patient and physician is as much a placebo as the pill given as placebo. You may argue that the procedure is as unnecessary as the pill, but that is a different argument from calling the procedure a placebo.

Physicians have to face the patient with abdominal pain who insists on an operation "to find out what is wrong," which usually means "to find out if I have a cancer." I believe that the proper question to ask such a patient is, "Well, supposing we explored you and found no cancer. How long would it take before you started worrying again?" To operate on such a patient is not to advise an operation as a placebo, but to make an error. Discussion is not furthered by calling such an approach placebic.

Indeed the economist could argue that treating some complaints first, with active drug or placebo, and investigating only those patients who failed to improve, might benefit the economy by reducing the cost of medical care.[30] The only problem such an economist might have is in fixing the charges for the placebo, if it is true that the more expensive the placebo, the more effective it is. That is an assumption which I have not seen proven.

Against the trifling cost of a medication must be put the much larger cost of diagnostic investigation, and more important, the inconvenience or discomfort of the procedure. The relief that comes to a physician and patient alike when pain is assuaged by a simple exchange is cheap indeed.

The Impure Placebo

Nevertheless a strong argument can be made against the use of the impure placebo, the drug which might be effective for one disorder or process but which is being used for another. Many currently marketed drugs probably work as impure placebos. Nader reported that 607 available drugs were no more effective than a placebo; 1.1 billion dollars worth of prescriptions were for drugs considered ineffective so far by the FDA. Clearly such drugs bring side effects with them, and although they assuage the physician's feelings about what he is doing, they bring more harm than good. Antibiotics used for colds of-

30. Fuchs, V., *Who shall live?* New York: Basic, 1974, p. 125.

fer one example of the impure placebo improperly used, for they bring more potential harm than good. Yet use of an impure placebo may protect the physician against a malpractice suit.

DIAGNOSTIC OBJECTIONS

Masking Disease

Another argument arrayed against the placebo is that it will relieve pain of serious origin so thoroughly that the doctor will be deluded into looking no further. In this way a disease which might have been treated will go unrecognized too long. The underlying belief seems to run that a disease which is found early can be treated better and more effectively than one which is discovered late. That makes common sense, but it depends upon the delay and upon the disease. There is very little convincing evidence that a *short* diagnostic delay affects the outcome of most diseases, except in malpractice courts.[31] No competent physician would deal with abdominal pain of sudden onset, for example, by other than emergency diagnostic tests and even an operation. But abdominal pain of some months or years duration might be another matter.

It does happen, very rarely, that treatment with an active drug before any diagnostic tests are carried out, masks disease. For example, giving H2 blockers to a patient with new dyspepsia may temporarily relieve even the pain of gastric cancer. This is rare, though I have seen a woman of thirty-three in whom the diagnosis of gastric cancer had been delayed for as much as nine months because her symptoms so completely responded to H2 blockade therapy.

To some extent commentators on these matters display more respect for medical practice than do physicians themselves. The questions that have to be asked are (1) whether a good response to a placebo has ever put off diagnostic studies for very long, or (2) whether, for most diseases, earlier detection in the asymptomatic person ever leads to a better outcome. Many people believe this, but the medical evidence is not so convincing that a specific diagnosis will be delayed enough so that the patient (not to mention the doctor) will get into trouble.

Detection bias. Detection bias is a problem. There is ordinarily no sharp line between when a disease begins and when it can be detected. To some extent what looks like a lifespan prolonged after early detection of diseases is the result of detecting the disease at an earlier stage

31. Spiro, H. M., Delayed diagnosis of disease, *JAMA* 233:2258, 1985.

than before. For example, primary biliary cirrhosis used to be a disease of middle-aged and elderly women. It ran a chronic but relatively short-lived course because it was recognized only late in its evolution. The development of a relatively specific blood test for biliary cirrhosis, detecting mitochondrial antibodies, allowed the detection of the disease in many young people, years before they developed any symptoms at all. The disease picture therefore changed from a short-lived but chronic problem of old women who suffered from jaundice and itching (because that is what brought them to attention) to one equally characteristic of much younger women who had no complaints at all, except as knowing about their "problem" might have made them more attentive to any symptom.

The increasing automation of laboratory tests, therefore, is responsible for an apparent change in the clinical presentation of primary biliary cirrhosis. It is now commonly a disease of younger women who do not know that they have signs, or that their minor complaints are even its symptoms, until the doctor tells them. Therefore primary biliary cirrhosis now looks like a much milder disease than it did fifteen or twenty years ago. The disease itself has not changed, but the physician's ability to make the diagnosis before symptoms develop has been markedly enhanced.

Delayed diagnosis? I can find no evidence that placebos are powerful enough to delay for very long the manifestations of any disease; if such a delay exists, I do not know how long that delay may be. If it proves to be very long, then the power of the placebo will deserve even greater admiration. It is surprising how commentators who are not physicians seem to assume that every complaint must have an objective cause, or should be proven not to, and that a delay of days or even several weeks to await the effect of any treatment may injure the patient's prospects for recovery. Physicians may have taught their lessons entirely too well. As far as I can tell no physician who has looked at this issue has had the same concern as the layman about delayed diagnosis from using a placebo. It is almost as if physicians all agree that placebos help pain, diminish suffering, but do little to relieve the serious manifestations of "organic" disease.

I do need to emphasize that what I have been talking about is the relief of pain and not the relief of other kinds of symptoms. With pain I include anxiety, depression, concern, foreboding, and the like. Other complaints require investigation, and what I have been writing about should not be taken to mean otherwise. For example, the person complaining of rectal bleeding clearly should never be put off with placebo therapy, nor even reassurances or symptomatic management without thorough investigation. Even though its source may prove to be the ubiquitous but innocuous hemorrhoid, the likelihood of a serious origin to rectal bleeding is enough to brook no diagnostic delay. Even in the matter of pain I dare not suggest that chest pain or acute pain of any origin be treated first with a placebo or with compassion. That is why a physician must make such decisions. But I am trying to emphasize that pain is what a placebo relieves. More objective suggestions of disease must be investigated by more usual medical means.

Therapeutic Detours

The final argument against placebos is what might be called the therapeutic detour. Even if placebos work, they may block the efforts of the patient to get at the cause of his problem. In its baldest form the argument holds that a placebo which relieves pain keeps the patient from seeing a psychiatrist, or at least readjusting his life as much as possible to reduce pain and suffering. Here such observers must ask whether they may be urging their own values on the patient. Many patients resist seeking psychological help, but that psychiatric help may prove so wrenching, expensive, or unpredictably beneficial that, weighed in the balance, the expedient of trying a placebo, with the aforementioned disclaimers, seems much easier.

There is another problem, of course. People often deny illness or disease, the new onset of troubles. A patient who has finally screwed up his courage enough to seek a doctor's help and who gets a placebo may take refuge in such reassurance and not return when his complaints are not assuaged. "The doctor said I'm OK," he may tell anxious relatives.

It is also argued that a pill which gives relief, even if it is a placebo, will accustom the patient to rely upon medication for other disorders, to look for a magical potion for every problem. This is a serious argument without a good answer. Giving placebos could promote drug-taking and dependence on medication. I can only respond that faith in medication has such a long history that it seems unlikely to be strengthened any more than it currently is. One has only to look at the host of over-the-counter medications currently advertised to realize how widespread is faith in a pill. The physician's use of placebos is the potential drop in the bucket.

Placebo as "Nocecibo"

One other argument against the placebo is that it can cause harm, in which case it is called a nocecibo. There are two ways in which this happens, one by unintended side effects such as those of antibiotics and the other by way of conditioned responses which lead to pathophysiological effects. If the patient has had bad experiences with drugs before, they will be reinvoked by a conditioned response, in the nocecibo effect.

So great is the belief in the dark side to the placebo effect that it has been used as an argument against fully informed consent, in the fear that "explicit suggestion of possible adverse effects causes subjects to experience these effects."[32] The well-known authors of that suggestion, "Informed consent may be hazardous to health", suggest that "the possible consequences of suggested symptoms range from minor annoyance to, in extreme cases, death."

The very cogent point has also been made that the person who spends too much time worrying about the complications of a diagnostic procedure or of a drug, however rare those complications, may not be in a "positive frame of mind." Therefore he may not mobilize the healing processes of the body as effectively as someone whom a more paternalistic approach has protected against undue concern. It will take much work to prove this intuitively sensible suggestion. As I have already suggested, this seems theoretically possible but unlikely. Impure placebos, such as antibiotics, however, can produce harmful effects.

Malpractice and the Placebo

The patient's reactions. We must ask, of course, what the patient's reaction will be to finding out that he has been given a placebo, particularly one which has not been helpful. In my account so far, I have discussed the response of his pain, but not the patient's personal reaction.

"You mean", he might react if the pain is not helped, "you gave me a sugar pill and charged me for your services? What kind of fool do you take me for? Do you think me a child?" It is not easy for me to imagine giving a professor of molecular biology at Yale a sugar pill for his pain without at least telling him what I am doing. I fear that in such circumstances anger, resentment, hostility, and a whole host of emotions might lead to a lawsuit or at least to changing physicians.

General distrust of doctors. Bok suggests that widespread placebo-giving might lead to a good deal of perplexity and uncertainty about the medical profession.[33] The physician might well ask himself whether in giving a placebo to a patient he has treated that patient too much as a child. Here I reaffirm that the physician should never give

32. Loftus, E. F., and Fries, J. F., Informed consent may be hazardous to health, *Science* 204:6, 1979.

33. Bok, *Lying*.

a placebo as a fraud, that is, one should never give a placebo without telling the patient at the least that you are giving him something which is not known to be active but rather something which the physician thinks may help the patient for reasons that are difficult to explain. I have discussed the spirit in which the placebo should be given elsewhere and whether so doing is misrepresenting the situation. Still, it is probable that some patients will react angrily to the discovery that they have been given a placebo, particularly if it is expensive. Yet in practice, the physician rarely finds a patient who gets upset, perhaps because patients are so rarely told what has happened.

I confess that I have used the placebo as a symbol, that the placebo served as a metaphor for communication, for contact, for *giving* to the patient. In our sophisticated society with scientific medicine, the only placebos that will be tolerated—if for no other reasons than to avoid a lawsuit—will be the impure placebo, one with some action creditable toward relieving the patient's complaints and treating the system, ostensibly their source. No current physician can seriously justify complete fraud or utter magic and most physicians have to have some respect for their own scientific background. Few physicians in 1986 give the kinds of sugar pills that the previous generation provided, but physicians give antibiotics or vitamin B12 or other injections to reassure the patient, and, alas, sometimes because they get paid for giving the shots. Some rely on diagnostic tests or operations. Reassurance can come in other ways, and just as we have educated patients in this half-century to expect scientific medicine and every available diagnostic test, it seems probable that in the future people can be educated to expect less in the way of diagnostic studies and more in the way of comfort.

Malpractice suits. Curiously enough, there have been few legal rulings on the use of the placebo and whether a doctor runs the risk of a malpractice suit when he prescribes one for a patient.[34] In the past the placebo aroused little interest among lawyers, probably because most patients never found out they had been given one, so that case law based on precedent and decision by judges about the practice has not been erected.

Judges and lawyers will be thinking more about the placebo for a number of reasons: many more physicians practice in groups now and team medicine is almost the norm in hospitals. Awareness that a patient is being given a placebo is much less likely to be kept secret among so many people. Moreover pharmacists may be, as Kapp suggests, increasingly reluctant to deceive their customers about their

34. Kapp, U. B., Placebo therapy and the law: Prescribe with care, *Am. J. L. Med.* 8:371, 1982.

prescriptions. Conceivably they might even tell them that they are getting sugar pills, particularly if a third-party pays the bills. At any event there are so many links in the chain between physician and patient that the placebo transaction is ever more likely to become known and the patient to sue for deception, fraud, or even malpractice.

Jurcich v. General Motors. In *Jurcich* v. *General Motors Corporation* in the Missouri Court of Appeals in 1976 lawyers sought $5,000 actual damages and $250,000 punitive damages because the plaintiff had been given placebos for back pain on a number of occasions.[35] Emil Jurcich had worked for the Fisher Body Division of General Motors. Crossing the assembly line on June 5, he was hit in the back by a "seat press being pushed down the assembly line." At the plant dispensary, where he went to complain of lower back pain, he was given an ice-pack and a muscle relaxant. On subsequent visits on June 10, 20, and several times after July 6, the nurse in the dispensary gave him "a sugar pill," telling him it was "a pain pill." As a direct result of this deception Mr. Jurcich claimed he continued to have pain in his back, which would not have been the case if he had been given pain-relievers rather than placebo. Over the subsequent six months he sought care elsewhere, was put in traction, and given heat, massage, and exercise. Finally, three years later, in 1971, Mr. Jurcich received 20 percent permanent partial disability. At the Workman's Compensation Commission hearings which granted him that disability he learned for the first time that he had received placebos and brought suit.

The court ruled that the prescribing of placebos was a recognized form of treatment and quoted some witnesses who had testified by deposition. Dr. K. Fritsch testified: "No. You never tell anyone if you are going to give them a placebo, then you know it won't work. You are hoping that you will fool him." The court did not hold that giving placebos worsened the patient's pain and emphasized that pain and suffering are recoverable as damages only when there has been a personal injury, and the pain and suffering is the proximate result of the defendant's wrongful act. That was not the case simply because Mr. Jurich had been given placebos. Nor was there evidence, since the case was being tried on grounds of fraud, that the patient had suffered a monetary loss as the result of the placebo. The trial court's ruling was upheld in the appellate court.

Kapp, a lawyer who has considered the legal implications of placebo-giving very thoroughly, suggests several bases for suing a physician who gives out placebos without telling the patient what he is doing.[36]

35. *Jurcich* v. *General Motors Corp.*, 539 S.W. 2d 595 (Mo App. 1976)
36. Kapp, Placebo therapy.

Fraud. Fraud supplies the first grounds: one of the elements of fraud is "a statement, a guilty silence, or a concealment," especially in circumstances in which there is a fiduciary relationship between two people. A patient might sue a physician on grounds that he would have gone to another physician if he had known his doctor was prescribing a placebo. Whether knowing he was getting a placebo would have made any difference to the patient's care or to the outcome of his complaint is arguable, and the problem of determining damages is fraught with difficulty. In a few cases placebo-giving has been considered grounds for fraud—a tort—in lawyers' language. Judges have commented in such suits that malpractice would have provided better grounds since it is hard to prove the requisite damages which can be recompensed by money to the patient who has been given a placebo. No one, so far, seems to have discussed the question of whether giving an impure placebo, one with some pharmacological action, however irrelevant to the complaint, might provide a defense.

Of course third-party payers, who have to pay for a placebo they might judge to be worthless, could conceivably bring suit, particularly if the pharmacist charged more than a minimal amount for the "drug." In a unique twist, I have heard that people who have been given an inactive powder instead of illicit drugs have threatened to sue for fraud.

Informed consent. The second, and more likely, grounds for suit might be on an informed consent basis, or more properly on the lack of informed consent. People have the right to know what is being done to them; giving a placebo without telling the patient about it is certainly open to the informed consent argument. The problem in winning such a suit, however, would lie in showing that harm befell the patient taking the placebo.

Injury. The third basis for suing a physician for giving a placebo might be malpractice, to compensate the patient for injuries suffered through the fault of the physician. Proving injury is likely only if the patient had suffered a negative placebo reaction, but most evidence suggests that such an event is unlikely. However, claiming that the use of a placebo prevented or delayed more appropriate treatment which would have been effective in detecting or arresting the disorder under treatment might well lead to a successful suit for malpractice. Kapp invokes the "doctrine of rescue" to suggest that a "liability is created" by physicians who give a placebo and so prevent the patient from tentatively seeking out more adequate care. The physician who gives a placebo which relieves the patient runs very little risk, but if the placebo does not help, then the physician might well be held liable for not changing treatment once it was clear that the placebo was ineffective. The physician, or an institution dispensing placebos as part of a controlled clinical trial, is presumably protected by the original informed consent laying out the double-blind nature of the trial. But once the outcome of the trial becomes clear, for whatever reason, ethical and legal considerations demand an end to the trial even if its continuance would make the statistical basis stronger.

Breach of contract. Breach of contract, the implied promise by the physician to be honest, is the fourth category, but one which Kapp suggests provides only a relatively weak basis for a malpractice suit.[37]

Defenses

No injury. Reviewing the potential defenses against being sued for giving a placebo, Kapp suggests that the first—and no doubt the strongest and most often used—defense lies in the claim that no damage has occurred because no injury has been done. To prove liability the plaintiff has to show that he has been injured. Unless the patient can show he has suffered an adverse reaction to the placebo or that his condition worsened during the time he was taking the placebo, it will be difficult to prove damages. The courts, however, have occasionally held just that opinion.

Accepted practice. A second defense will depend upon showing that other physicians use placebos, that there is no negligence. The accepted practice of physicians includes giving placebos.

Therapeutic privilege. The third and chief defense so far used has been the justification that placebos do alleviate the complaint of many patients and that they are, therefore, permitted under the "doctrine of therapeutic privilege." If, in the professional judgment of a physician, telling the patient that he has given him a placebo would complicate or hinder treatment, or just upset the patient enough to cause psychological harm, it has been held permissible to proceed with treatment without informed consent. It has been common physician opinion that the beneficial effect of placebos depends upon deception; many physicians might argue that full disclosure would lessen the relief from a placebo. On the other hand, Kapp emphasizes, such a so-called privilege of necessity has been limited to emergencies. Once the patient has improved, then full disclosure of the fact that the patient is getting a placebo should take place. To avoid any possi-

37. Ibid.

ble suit a physician should probably consult with a colleague to get an independent written assessment of his proposal to give a placebo under the doctrine of therapeutic privilege. That seems like such a farfetched notion to most practitioners that it may be impractical. One of my friends has asked whether he should call the consultant while the patient is dressing before prescribing a placebo. (Whether just getting that second opinion might itself have placebo effect, every practicing physician will wonder.)

Solutions

Waiver. A patient has the right to waive his right to all information; such a waiver can be implied by his demeanor, facial expression, behavior, and the like. A waiver of information need not be explicit, but I believe that this idea needs more study and testing by the courts.

Incomplete disclosure. Kapp suggests "incomplete disclosure" as the way out of the problem. A patient can contract with his physician to permit the physician to withhold from the patient any "anti-therapeutic information." The patient in effect says to his physician, "You are the doctor. Tell me what I need to know. I trust you and if you don't want to tell me something that you think will hurt me, don't. I am in your hands." That sounds like an explicit rephrasing of the old-fashioned, previously implicit physician-patient relationship. How much the patient needs to know can be decided by the physician once he has received permission from the patient. But such a plan will seem overly paternalistic to many.

It seems increasingly likely that physicians run a risk of suit for prescribing placebos, but it also seems likely that it still would be difficult to prove that the placebo was harmful unless a diagnosis of some serious disorder was thereby delayed. What a significant delay might be has to be argued. I maintain that delaying the diagnosis of gastric cancer, for example, for ten days or so to test the benefit of H2 blockers for new-onset dyspepsia is blameless, and indeed praiseworthy. It might be much more difficult to convince a judge that a month's delay was equally guiltless. An impure placebo aiming at the symptoms to be treated may prove to be the best possible defense, however unreasonable it may seem from the purely medical standpoint. Of course giving an impure placebo brings a greater risk of real harm to the patient, as Bok pointed out. The next few years should bring more judgments to bear on those matters.

Returning to the use of placebo as dummy, we must ask whether it is ethical or even reasonable to compare a new drug against a placebo in a double-blind controlled trial, if another known drug has already proven beneficial. That is, should a new drug be compared to an inactive placebo, or should it be compared to a drug known, by previous trials, to be beneficial? From the scientist's standpoint, comparing new drugs to ones which were already accepted might lead to the accepting of a number of drugs which "work," but which may not be more effective than a placebo. From the legal standpoint, clearly the patients who receive a placebo might well sue if they suffered harm from receiving placebo rather than a known active drug. Yet such considerations have led to all kinds of complications, as Dollery has pointed out.[38] Does a patient who has a stroke on a placebo during a trial have the right to sue his doctor, the organization running the trial, or society? Moreover, if a drug is shown to reduce the risk of a stroke by one-third in a high-risk group, should the patients who receive the controlled drug be compensated, only a third of them, or which third? These are not issues which we will answer, but physicians should be aware of them.

What about the use of placebo in controlled trials? We have already discussed the problem of whether a patient receives a placebo in a drug trial and who is therefore deprived of the benefit of an effective currently available drug has been injured from a moral standpoint. There are legal considerations. The patient whose ulcer bleeds while he is taking a placebo might argue that had he known of the potential consequences, he might not have joined the trial. Yet society does need such trials. One way out, Dollery suggests, is to compensate persons who take part in trials because they are serving the public good as much or more than their own. Yet the difficulties of deciding upon the amount of compensation, at least ahead of time, seem very great. He asks: "Suppose a large trial showed that aspirin reduced the risk of a fatal myocardial infarction by one-third in a high risk group of patients? Would all the patients in the control group be compensated or only a third and, if so, which third? Or would all receive a third of the compensation that they might have received, if the treatment had been completely effective in the other group?"

Placebos represent a form of altruistic deception which can be used to help, but should not be used only to deceive. The patient should know what is going on and the physician should not delude himself by attributing solely to himself too magical powers.

38. Dollery, C. T., A bleak outlook for placebos (and for science), *Europ. J. Clin. Pharmacol.* 15:219–21, 1979.

10

Analogies with the Placebo

Everyone can be influenced by someone else to some degree, directly or indirectly. The sick need help more than the healthy and are more susceptible to consolation. A comforting relationship between therapist and patient, regardless of any theory behind the therapist's ministrations, will lighten the patient's perceptions of his problems. That is what makes assessing and defining alternative medicine so difficult.

Moreover, alternative medicine is nothing new. Goddard concluded in 1899 that

> cures by mind-cure exist, but are in no respect different from those now officially recognized in medicine as cures by suggestion. . . . We have traced the mental element through primitive medicine and folk medicine of today, patent medicine, and witchcraft. We are convinced that it is impossible to account for the existence of these practices, if they did not cure disease, and that if they cure disease, it must have been the mental element that was effective.[1]

It is not easy to arrive at a definition of alternative medicine, for the term covers most forms of therapy that do not fit into current medical practices. Sometimes alternative therapy is given by lay people and sometimes by cult practitioners. Physicians who practice alternative medicine usually call it "holistic" medicine. I use *alternative medicine* to mean any therapeutic program which defines itself as outside the mainstream of practice and which aims in some unconventional

---

1. Goddard, H. H., The effect of mind on body as evidenced by faith cures, *Amer. J. Psychol.* 10 (1894), quoted by James, W., *The varieties of religious experience*, New York: Modern Library, (n.d.,) p. 95.

manner at relieving symptoms. Alternative therapy can be given by unlicensed practitioners outside the medical profession or can be given as unconventional therapy by physicians in a sometimes unconventional manner. Of course, as Paul Wolpe has reminded me, what is conventional in one culture is unconventional in another; acupuncture offers a good example.[2] Such alternatives to high-technology drug-based medicine include hypnosis, acupuncture, homeopathy, herbal medicine, faith healing, and many other approaches. Major distinctions between alternative and orthodox medicine lie in the expressed aim of alternative practitioners to treat the whole person rather than a specific symptom or a disease, and in the unorthodox therapeutic approaches. Many mainstream practitioners, of course, also treat the whole person without considering themselves beyond the pale, but for the most part they focus on disease. To some extent alternative medicine aims at health rather than sickness, and I hope to show that it helps illness not disease.

In reading about alternative medicine, keep in mind how important it is to distinguish relief of illness from cure of disease. Anthropologists or holistic practitioners are not always better at such distinction than medical practitioners.

I ignore, for the most part, witchcraft and voodoo. I distinguish between making a sick person well, which is analogous to the therapeutic placebo, and making a well person sick, as in voodoo.

The shortcomings of modern medical practice with so much emphasis on disease and perhaps too little on the person provide one reason for a revival of interest in nontraditional modes of treatment. If it is true that 70 to 90 percent of all "complaints" are now handled outside the usual medical system, then the trend over the past seventy-five years to try to put all medical care in the hands of licensed medical practitioners is being reversed informally by the renewed emphasis on self-care in what its proponents claim is a "nonbureaucratic" way.[3] The dominance of the orthodox physician, refreshed by the Flexner report and sustained by the real successes of scientific medicine (and celebrated by professional organizations), has been challenged, and may be yielding a little to holistic medicine, and various forms of nonphysician care. We physicians may condemn such alternative activities as irrational and find an unfair parallel with popular interest in demonology, but such supernaturalism is part of the long tradition of Romanticism challenging Rationalism, the Counter-Enlightenment after the Enlightenment. Even educated people with

2. Wolpe, P., Personal communication, 1984.
3. Levin, L. S., and Idlen, E. L., Self-care in health, *Ann. Rev. Pub. Health* 4:181–201, 1983.

cancer will seek out unorthodox practitioners who emphasize nutrition and personal responsibility along with physical fitness and an improved mental attitude, and who provide more personal warmth than some technologically oriented practitioners.[4]

In Britain matters have moved even further: a campaign may be mounted to recognize alternative practitioners, partly to give them status and partly to protect the public. Indeed Inglis tells us that the Council of Europe has set up a committee to look into alternative medicine, "in view of the frequency with which sick people nowadays seek help from non-conventional practitioners, this phenomenon can no longer be regarded as a medical side issue. . . . It must reflect a genuine public need."[5]

Alternative medical practices deserve the attention of the medical profession rather than our instinctive disavowal, but we must look at them as critically and rationally as we examine claims for the placebo. The dismaying enthusiasm for the occult displayed in books, movies, and newspaper items provide the atavistic counterpart to some popular treatments of disease. Yet such general hysteria (I can only call it that) must be telling us physicians to widen our definitions of disease, to expand our metaphors of disease and the range of our activities. I would give the ear emphasis equal to the eye; now diagnosis depends only on the eye, but it could, in many instances, depend equally well upon listening to the patient, on the ear, so to speak.

Healing is a term we will encounter repeatedly in surveying alternative medicine. It has enormous vogue at the moment in nonmedical circles, but healing is not a word which physicians use very often anymore. Cassell uses it in his fine advice in *The Healer's Art*, but curiously he never defines it: "I used the word 'healer' and suddenly saw that I had no idea what it really meant."[6] He uses the word *disease* as I have used it, and discusses illness as the reaction to disease influenced by culture and psyche. For Cassell doctors cure disease, healers help illness, but for him illness is becoming helpless, like a child, being fearful, fearful of death: "The spector of helplessness looms" (p. 166). The healer is a magical omnipotent figure for Cassell, who would lend the fearful patient his own confidence, to bridge the world of the sick. His healer is confident, charismatic, a source of omnipotence, who returns control to the sick, or who gives permission like a parent:

> The doctor's sense of omipotence is an important part of his function as a healer, something he cannot disown. But omnipo-

4. Tobias, J. S., and Tattersall, M. H., Doing the best for the cancer patient, *Lancet* 1:35–37, 1985.

5. Inglis, B., Alternative medicine: Is there a need for registration? *Lancet* 1:95–96, 1985.

6. Cassell, E. J., *The Healer's Art*, New York: Penguin, 1976, p. 14.

tence, like all magical gifts, is double-edged and dangerous; it can strengthen as well as harm its possessor and its receiver. The doctor's feeling of omnipotence can foster dependency, making a despot of the doctor and a child of the patient, or it can give the patient courage to learn control and free himself from fear. (p. 163)

Frank, whose influential writings I have found very helpful, avoids a definition in his book *Persuasion and Healing*.[7] Healing seems to be "measures which combat anxiety and arouse hope," which "strengthen his sense of self-worth" (pp. 65 and 53). For Frank is a psychiatrist, after all, and emphasizes that religious healing shows "the profound influence of emotions on health and suggests that anxiety and despair can be lethal, confidence and hope, life-giving." I do not make these comments to criticize either Cassell or Frank, both of whom have strongly influenced my thinking, but simply to emphasize the problems that modern physicians of the orthodox variety have in using the term *healing*. For both, healing affects illness. If we hope to arrive at a synthesis of psychosomatic medicine as that aspect of disease which looks at the whole person, attempts—in Frank's and Cassell's terms —to "heal" him, clarifying what we mean by healing will be the first step.

In the *OED* I find that as a transitive verb, *heal* means "to make whole or sound in bodily condition; to free from disease or ailment, restore to health or soundness; to cure (of a disease or wound)." Another definition is "to perform or effect a cure; to restore to soundness." And yet another definition, more figurative, "is to restore a person from some evil condition or affection (as sin, grief, disrepair, unwholesomeness, danger, destruction) to save, purify, cleanse, repair, mend." Clearly we are talking about different processes when we talk about healing just as, Davies points out[8], we must distinguish between *faith* and ignorant *credulity*, a belief founded on weak or insufficient evidence.

Healing sometimes makes claims that the modern physician is loathe to set for himself: "I dress the wound, God heals it."[9]

Healing is a term with implications that the physician seldom wishes to avow. Holistic medicine makes claims for healing, and so do some charlatans, but for the physician *cure* is a more comfortable word. That has to do, I think, with his looking only at disease. Healing brings a connotation of curing from within, as in "the wound heals," a

7. Frank, J. D., *Persuasion and healing*, New York: Schocken, 1963.

8. Davies, G., The hands of the healer: Has faith a place? *J. Med. Ethics* 6:185–89, 1980.

9. Pare, A., "I treated him, God cured him," quoted as such in *Bartlett's familiar quotations*, 14th ed., Boston: Little Brown, 1968, p. 187.

connotation of a return to health or wholeness that means more than the physician thinks he can claim.

Dean, a holistic practitioner, suggests that healing, broadly defined, rests on (1) nature's self-reparative processes, (2) suggestion, (3) the therapeutic personality of the healer, (4) the expectant faith of the patient, and (5) "an interchange of energy" between healer and patient: "To the extent the therapist is able to envision and call forth healing and wholeness within his patients, he is manifesting in action those qualities that are within himself."[10] It should be clear that people use the term *healing* in so many different ways that agreement is unlikely. We just need to keep these different usages in mind.

Studies of medical practices in other cultures provide a prudent distance for looking at alternative medicine. If we can recognize how other cultures regard disease and disability, we may find that Western biomedical models do not fit all human complaints.

MEDICAL ANTHROPOLOGY

Landy defines medical anthropology as "the study of human confrontations with disease and illness, and of the adaptive arrangements (that is, medicines and medical systems) made by human groups for dealing with these ever-present and panhuman dangers."[11] Although disease is universal, aside from genetic and environmental influences, people in different cultures express their diseases and disabilities in vastly different ways, depending upon the general indoctrination into a consensus of what an illness is and what causes it—or just as important—what it is fitting to feel and to discuss. An unpleasant bodily sensation will be interpreted by people quite differently depending upon their social and cultural matrix. How pain is interpreted, for example, will determine the kind of help that will be sought; different kinds of practitioners will give different explanations; and the declared disease will be treated differently in different societies. Alcohol use is a common example. Plato's discussion of drinking parties as a "great contribution to education if it is done correctly"[12] would not have gone unchallenged in late-nineteenth-century Indiana.

Anthropologists and sociologists teach physicians to look at the social and even symbolic dimensions of how an illness is defined.[13] If

10. Sampson, R., Healing in the treatment of modern medicine, *Somatics* 1978:8–14 (Dean quoted by)

11. Landy, D., ed., *Culture, disease, and healing.* New York: MacMillan, 1977, p. 1.

12. *The laws of Plato,* T. L. Pangle, trans., New York: Basic, 1980, p. 21.

13. Moerman, D. E., Anthropology of symbolic healing, *Current Anthropol.* 20:59-80, 1979; Moerman, D. E., Physiology and Symbols: The anthropological implications

his society expects a person to perform certain basic tasks, there has to be a way for a sick person to have his status as "sick" accepted by society. How that is done will vary depending upon the notion of disease. Friedson has emphasized the legitimatizing role of the physician in Western culture in defining the patient as sick so that the patient is freed of responsibilities and can sever his connections without stigma.[14] (That the physician is more likely to accept as sick the patient with a disease that he can see, more than the patient with only a complaint, is another matter.) Being sick, to some extent, limits your role in society, legitimizes not working, and has a host of other symbolic functions.

Anthropological studies of illness and disease contribute to the understanding of the placebo effect, and of medical practice generally, in at least three ways: (1) concrete examples from other cultures can make physicians aware of how the models of disease that a society holds affect how patients and physicians define disabilities and complaints and how they react to them; (2) anthropologists describe phenomena such as voodoo or witchcraft which need analysis and reflection, although they cannot always be explained; (3) finally, observations of folk medicine offer clues to the physician-patient relationship in the Western world[15] and help to illuminate the placebo effect.[16]

Anthropological studies of healing practices in non-Western and in preindustrial or premodern cultures have stressed how much the concept of disease varies from one culture to another. They thus prove a salutary antidote to Western reification of disease and provide a mirror for physicians to view what they do from outside.[17] Kleinman, Eisenberg, and Good have underlined the contributions of anthropological studies to the distinctions between disease and illness.[18] The biological model, so successful in the management of disease, should be linked to "ethnomedical" and "other medical" models, they suggest. Such a link forged by teachers in the medical schools might help to bring about changes in general perspectives on health, sickness,

of the placebo effect, in *The anthropology of Medicine*, ed. L. Romanucci-Ross, D. E. Moerman, and L. R. Tancredi, New York: Praeger, 1983.

14. Freidson, E., Disability as social deviance, in D. Roeschmeyer, Doctors and lawyers: A comment on the theory of the profession, in *Medical men and their work*, E. Freidson and J. Lorber, eds., Chicago: Aldine-Atherton, 1972.

15. Ibid, Fabrega, H., The need for an ethnomedical science, *Science* 189:969–75, 1975, Hahn, R. A., and Kleinman, A., Biomedical practice and anthropological theory, *Ann. Rev. Anthropol.* 12:305–33, 1983.

16. Fabrega, The need for an ethnomedical science.

17. Hahn and Kleinman, Biomedical practice and anthropological theory.

18. Kleinman, A., Eisenberg, L., and Good, B., Culture, illness, and care-clinical lessons from anthropologic and cross-cultural research, *Ann. Intern. Med.* 88:251–58, 1978.

and health care. As it is, few medical schools have any course in medical anthropology, and very few teachers in medical schools that I know are even aware of the professional organization, The Society for Medical Anthropology. Too many physicians remain unaware of medical anthropological observations and if they knew about them, might feel uncomfortable at finding themselves compared even fleetingly to witch doctors.[19]

Personalistic versus Naturalistic Systems

Systems which have an inherent rational basis, however flawed it may appear to Westerners, should be distinguished from those which rest on purely supernatural explanations. (Social scientists suggest that all healing systems have a rational basis, but that sometimes the rational foundation has been lost and a supernatural explanation remains to justify actions which once had reasons.) In some societies, religion and medical practice are inseparable; in others they are as separate as in the West. It may be pertinent to recall the distinctions that sociologists make between culture and society.[20] Medicine as cultural system is a way of thinking, a way of conceptualizing health and disease, and of making diagnoses and giving therapy. As a culture medicine teaches its students a single mode of perception. As a social system, something which will not detain us in looking at the placebo, medicine has a set of hierarchical organized roles with division of labor and institutional structures. For present purposes we are interested only in the culture and how that affects the views of disease, disability and illness.

Foster has usefully divided the way that cultures deal with the cause of illness: (1) in the *personalistic* system an agent, which may be human, nonhuman, or supernatural, intervenes to cause disease or pain; (2) in a *naturalistic* system natural forces or conditions are deemed responsible for disease.[21] In the naturalistic system imbalance of body elements, such as the classic humors of the Greeks or the *yin* or *yang* of the Asians, leads to disease. Foster suggests that many contemporary naturalistic systems have a "hot-cold" dichotomy, disease being explained by excessive cold or heat entering the body. "Feed a cold and starve a fever," many grandmothers' advice, to some

19. Prince, R. H., Psychotherapy as the manipulation of endogenous healing mechanisms: A transcultural survey, *Transcultural Psychiatry Research Review* 13:115–33, 1976.

20. Roeschemeyer, D., Doctors and lawyers: A comment on the theory of the profession, in *Medical men and their work*, E. Freidson, and J. Lorber, eds. Chicago: Aldine-Atherton, 1972.

21. Foster, G. M., Disease etiologies in non-western medical systems, *Amer. Anthropol.* 78:773–82, 1976.

extent suggests how this notion still finds a place in Western folk beliefs. In a study of poor blacks near Tucson Snow found that illness
was classified as "natural" or "unnatural"; natural illnesses are those
produced by the forces of nature acting on the person without suitable protection, whereas unnatural influences are personalistic, leading to diseases caused by witchcraft, "roots," and so forth.[22]

Personalistic explanations of disease are part of a "world view," a
comprehensive explanatory system, whereas a naturalistic system offers an explanation for illness and nothing more. An important consequence of the two systems, Foster suggests, is the different requirements for cure. In the personalistic system the shaman or priest or
witch doctor must have supernatural or magical skills to find out who
caused the disease. Once that is known, appropriate propitiation
leads to cure. Achilles was faced with the plague that was killing the
Greek soldiers,

> Rank and file
> sickened and died
> for the ill their chief had done
> in despising a man of prayer

He asked,

> Why all this anger of the God Apollo?
> Has he some quarrel with us for a failure
> in vows or hekatombs? Would mutton burned
> or smoking goat flesh make him lift the plague?[23]

Naturalistic systems require the more classical "doctor" who understands the origin of disease and can devise appropriate treatment. Examples from the naturalistic system offer useful parallels to the placebo. For the most part, however, I find the personalistic approach
less help in thinking about the placebo; someone may believe that he
is sick because he has been cursed and respond to a placebic intervention. Both systems lead to an "explanation" of disease, but the personalistic view is "nonphysiologic," much like old-fashioned hysteria,
whereas the naturalistic view, however mistaken, has an internal logic
like a "psychosomatic" complaint.

Naturalistic systems are more congenial to the modern physician as
that system sees diseases as arising from an imbalance of humors, of
hot and cold, or other principles. They require a rational, empirical
approach to their alleviation, whether it is through the diets of the
Greek physicians or the manipulations of the village healer. However

22. Snow, L. F., Folk medical beliefs and their implications for care of patients, *Ann.
Intern. Med.* 81:82–96, 1974.
23. Homer, *The Iliad*, trans. Robert Fitzgerald, New York: Anchor, 1974.

primitive they may be, naturalistic concepts have something in common with modern medical practice in their seemingly logical basis, no doubt refined by generations, more than the personalistic tradition which sees disease as the ill will of an outside agent.

Personalistic Systems

The personalistic system requires suppression of a rational approach to medical practice. The Western-trained physician is just unable to comprehend all that goes on with, or into, witchcraft and what it means, literally, to someone raised in that culture.

Witchcraft. The wide gulf between science and sorcery was not bridged some years ago in the *British Medical Journal*, when Dr. Konotey-Ahulu of Ghana voiced his disappointment at how Dr. Margaret Field, schoolteacher, physician, and psychiatrist, could have so accurately described the *juju* houses and fetish shrines of his tribe, taking photographs and making notes and yet so miss "the spiritual side of the whole thing."[24] She used "Western-European thought forms" as the standard, he complained, taking "demon possession" as only "hysterical exhibitionism." No Western physician could do otherwise; yet this modern African physician criticizes the persistent attempt to understand such phenomena by known psychological concepts, in Field's case largely Freudian ones.

Konotey-Ahulu gives us, ironically enough, the words of Pascal: "There are two excesses: to exclude reason, to admit nothing but reason." Concluding that science has no tools to probe spiritual things, he accepts them as "suprascientific." We can wonder at this, with a little shudder of horror, that an educated man can accept the reality of witchcraft, or more properly its effects. Yet from one point of view, is Konotey-Ahulu so different from the believing Western physician who accepts religious healing miracles? The witch doctor who removes a curse looks very little different, costume aside, from the clergyman casting out a devil, or an ancient Greek priest sacrificing hecatombs to Apollo. Whatever there is to such purported cures, more than endorphin stimulation, physicians have no better tools with which to examine the events than anyone else.

It may be arbitrary to exclude reports of personalistic intervention in disease from discussion of the placebo. Although such events deserve observation, classification, and analysis, I simply must set some limit on what is, at best, a discussion with trailing edges. Still, a few comments on faith healing may be in order.

24. Konotey-Ahulu, F., Personal view, *Brit. Med. J.* 1:1595, 1977.

Faith healing. We can use the definition of faith healing of Sir Henry Morris, a former president of the Royal College of Surgeons:

> In faith healing the suggestion is that cure will be worked by spiritual or divine power, especially if this power be appealed to at some particular place such as a sanctuary, the foot of an idol, a fountain or pool of water. . . . This divine power, or energy, is supposed to act by neutralizing or overcoming sickness, disease, and the ill consequences of accidents. The faith healer does not doubt the reality of matter or of diseases, but believes that he can draw upon a spiritual force to subdue or annihilate an existing evil.[25]

The very term is contentious, even for those who accept the phenomenon. A friend, an Anglo-Catholic priest, suggests that faith healing puts the locus of healing within the patient or the person who has the faith. That is where we physicians feel most comfortable putting it, all our physiological and other hypotheses about the placebo crediting the patient. My priestly friend prefers "spiritual healing" as giving credit to God. His is the personalistic view, where physicians like me take a naturalistic one. The conflict is as old as the Greeks, the conflict between the Hippocratic physicians who believed in science and the Aesculapians who helped through the mysteries of the temple. My friend may be right, but for now I use the term *faith*, implying that even though God may have created the endorphin system, man must wake it.

Faith healing in the Christian churches follows from James 5:14–15:

> Is any sick among you? Let him call for the Elders of the church; and let them pray over him, anointing him with oil in the name of the Lord: and the prayer of faith shall save the sick, and the Lord shall raise him up and if he has committed sins, they shall be forgiven him.

It is not my purpose to evaluate the miracles reported from time to time, though always curiously in out-of-the-way places and more often from the rural third world than the urban West. The greatest miracles, the most impressive cures, always seem to occur in primitive or rural conditions. Morris asked, "How came it about that the Alps and the Pyrenees . . . were so specially selected as the places at which these apparitions and miracles occur?"[26] He answered in relation to the "miracles" of the late nineteenth century which the Church did not

25. Morris, H., Suggestion in the treatment of disease, *Brit. Med. J.* 1:1457–66, 1910.
26. Morris, Suggestion.

accept: "Not entirely because France, Italy and Spain are the great Roman Catholic countries of the world, but chiefly, no doubt, for the reason that the inhabitants of the mountain districts are more impressionable to these manifestations."

What to the oncologist is only a chemotherapeutically induced remission may to the patient seem a miracle, but the matter is more than mere definition. Some sensitive, intelligent, and well-trained physicians believe that true miracles occur and that fractures can be healed, bleeding stopped, and many other matters beyond total scientific explanation can occur as a result of divine Grace.

I will ignore such events in agreement with Bonser's comments about faith healing, in which he quotes "'That dangerous field, placed between theology and medicine, that no one has dared thoroughly to explore.'"[27] I suspect that faith healers, spiritual healers, witch doctors, and others all achieve approximately the same results through the same final common pathway even though the stimuli may differ. No skepticism is intended, for I have not examined the issues. I believe that healers relieve pain and the emotional component of disease and that the healing touch and transference are not dissimilar, but I have not evaluated the problem. In his book *The Wounded Healer* Nouwen, a Catholic priest, talks of the healing minister:

> How does healing take place? Many words, such as care and compassion, understanding and forgiveness, fellowship and community have been used for the healing task. . . . It is healing because it takes away the false illusion that wholeness can be given by one to another. It is healing because it does not take away the loneliness and the pain of another, but invites him to recognize his loneliness in a level where it can be shared. . . . A minister is not a doctor whose primary task is to take away pain. Rather, he deepens the pain to a level where it can be shared.[28]

I believe that faith healing is not an alternative form of medicine, but that it provides a collaborative effort and that we must avoid an adversarial approach.

Davies comments that "skeptical scientists may then feel happy while believers of various kinds may simply feel that there is 'yet more light to break forth' on how nature (and the God of Nature) operates in what used to be called the *vis medicatrix naturae*."

The Emmanuel Movement. The Emmanuel Movement in Boston in the early twentieth century was just that sort of collaboration, as Osler

27. Bonser, W., The medical background of Anglo-Saxon England, London: Wellcome Historical Library, 1963, p. 211.

28. Nouwen, H. J., *The wounded healer.* Garden City: Image, 1972.

describes it. This faith healing movement, originated and supported by Dr. J. H. Pratt (for whom the Pratt Diagnostic Clinic was later named) undertook treatment of nervous troubles "by mental and spiritual agencies" along with a clergyman and a neurologist:

> Every applicant must first submit to diagnosis. If organic trouble is disclosed, he is not accepted as a patient. If the disease appears to be simply functional, the applicant is registered for treatment and passed on into the Rector's study. There he finds himself in an environment . . . which unlocks the hidden wholesomeness of his inner life and lead by rapid stages to complete recovery. . . .
>
> Where more is needed than the full self-revelation, in itself curative, and the prayer and godly counsel which succeeded, the patient is next invited to be seated in a reclining chair, taught to relax all his muscles, calmed by soothing words, and in a state of physical relaxation and mental quiet the unwholesome thoughts and the untoward symptoms are dislodged from his consciousness.[29]

This attempt to prevent as well as to cure functional ailments by looking at the whole patient does not sound unfamiliar today.

Christian Science. It may not be amiss to examine a series of comments on Christian Science which appeared in the *New England Journal of Medicine*. Of all the religious healing systems, Christian Science seems to be the most organized. Nathan Talbot, of that church, writes,

> Disease and physical suffering are in no sense caused or permitted by God, and that since they are profoundly alien to His creative purpose, it is wrong to resign oneself to them. . . . They believe that human beings are vastly more than biochemical mechanisms. . . .
>
> The basic Christian Science "diagnosis" of disease involves the conviction that whatever apparent form the disease assumes, it is in the last analysis produced by a radically limited and distorted view of the true spiritual nature and capacities of men and women.[30]

That is not too far from what we have been looking at, and the placebo might seem the secular equivalent of prayer. The problem comes in the apparent taking of part for whole, as so often is the case in alternative medicine.

In his discussion Talbot avoids the reasons why orthodox medical practice cannot be combined with using Christian Science as an adjunct:

29. Osler, W., The faith that heals, *Brit. Med. J.* 1:1470–72, 1910.

30. Talbot, N. A., The position of the Christian Science church *NEJM* 209:1641–44, 1983.

Some may think that spiritual healing as practiced by Christian Scientists is acceptable, or at least can do no harm, if employed as an
adjunct to medical treatment. The question that then arises is why
Christian Scientists believe as they do that their approach to healing cannot successfully be combined with medical treatment. To
them this view is not so much a matter of theoretical consistency as
one of practical and thoughtful concern for the welfare of patients.
As experience shows, the underlying thrusts of specific Christian
Science and medical treatment are so dissimilar that to seek healing
through both simultaneously is fair to neither of them.

He goes on to say that if a patient decides to turn to medical care, he is
released from Christian Science practitioners "in a supportive spirit
and without reproach."

Talbot's discussion was engendered by Rita Swan, once a devout
Christian Scientist.[31] After her son died of meningitis under the care
of a Christian Science practitioner, she became president of an organization called "Children's Health Care Is a Legal Duty." She seems
mainly to be—properly I think—against separating "prayer and support of patients" from the medical care system. The discussion which
followed led to many questions but no firm answers. In the recognition that many committed people can hardly discuss these issues, let
alone agree, I move on to other considerations.

Before doing so, however, let me note that one physician somewhat
impishly suggested a control trial of Christian Science versus antibiotics for childhood meningitis, predicting that such a trial probably
would never be carried out. That correspondent may not have read
Medawar's account of Francis Galton's "statistical inquiries into the efficacy of prayer," as a display of "science in its critical temper."[32]
Galton asked whether scientific evidence could be found for supposing that prayers were answered. In Britain the Queen was prayed for
weekly or daily on a national scale, but statistics did not suggest that
members of the Royal Family lived any longer than common people
as a result of prayers on their behalf. Nor could Galton find proof
that children of religious parents were less likely to be stillborn than
children of the professional classes (presuming of course that there
are fewer devout in that latter group). Finally, if the devout lived
longer than the skeptical, insurance companies would have learned to
charge religious believers a higher rate for an annuity because of their
longer life. Medawar relates that Galton comments that insurance

31. Swan, R., Faith healing, Christian Science, and the medical care of children,
NEJM 209:1639–41 1983.
32. Medawar, P. B., *Induction and intuition in scientific thought*, Philadelphia: American Philosophical Society, 1969.

companies "absolutely ignore prayer" in making confidential inquiries into the applicant's habits. On the basis of such statistical inquiry Galton could not conclude that prayers were answered. No doubt a similar investigation into the health and welfare of Christian Scientists and other people might be entirely feasible.

Naturalistic Systems

The shaman in various cultures has been studied exhaustively as the prototypical priest-doctor or medicine man. Let us turn from faith healing and the personalistic systems to some naturalistic views of disease as exemplified by the shaman to learn more about the effect of culture on the definition of disease, illness, and the treatments that seem appropriate. No matter how unusual the naturalistic concept, if it is internally coherent, its success in relieving symptoms should remind the practitioner that many logical schemes can seem to work even though from the standpoint of the biomedical purist they are flawed.

The shaman. In his study *The Shaman*, which compares shamanistic and Western methods of "healing," Spencer Rogers fails to distinguish between reports of healing and objective evidence of cure.[33] Like most anthropologists he accepts an "I-feel-better" from a person whose headache has been relieved by incantation as the equal of the same statement made by someone cured of pneumonia by penicillin. It is this confusion between the *objective* and the *subjective* that characterizes so many discussions of healing. For such reasons Rogers can pay particular attention to "the shaman's remarkable rate of success and to the dilemma faced by persons in developing countries who can choose either traditional healing methods or scientific medicine." Yet he has much to say about the profession of the shaman, his magic and healing methods, his contribution to understanding of psychotherapy and to "the causes and diagnosis of illness." Nowhere, however, despite some challenging comparisons of shamanistic and Western-style "doctoring" does the anthropologist-author give any attention to just what it is the shaman cures.

He defines a shaman as "a priest doctor who uses magic to cure the sick, to divine the hidden, and to control events that affect the welfare of the people" (p. ix). But he also adopts the notion that a shaman is a "professional in the field of the supernatural" (p. ix). Let us accept the limited and somewhat archaic definition of a professional as someone in one of the "service occupations that: 1) apply a systematic body of

33. Rogers, S. L., *The shaman, His symbols and his healing power*, Springfield: Thomas, 1982.

knowledge to problems which 2) are highly relevant to central values of the society."[34]

That makes the shaman a professional, however an orthodox physician may wince. If modern scholars require for a profession, in addition, self-policing and an abstract body of ideas, a shaman looks less like a professional than many others who claim that role: "The shaman may, at times, have recourse to methods that may be called *empirical science*—courses of action that are essentially naturalistic, but have not been repeatedly verified to the degree that they can be termed scientific."

It is of course a major problem that observation without even numeration or verification is equated by many observers of folk healing as equivalent to the more predictable sciences of modern medicine. Rogers is careful to emphasize that primitive, non-Western folk medicine is not an entity, but that each of many cultures has its own quite different doctrines or methods despite their "striking and unexplained similarities."

Comparing Western and primitive medicine, Rogers suggests how

the Western physician and the shaman both attempt to establish a logical explanation for the onset of any particular illness. . . . Each uses his own specialized approach towards the control of disease, and both approaches are logical. The western physician attacks the problem through an understanding of the parts of the human body machine: its cells, organs, and their functions. The shaman seeks the reason in the supernatural events: the breaking of taboos, magic spells, and the anger of gods. (p. 161)

As we turn to control of illness, in strict contrast to disease, a distinction which it must be emphasized again that Rogers—like most anthropologists—does not recognize or maintain, we can see, however, many parallels with Western medicine:

The shaman's first step in attempting to heal is to establish a thorough confidence on the part of the sufferer, his relatives, and other members of the community. They must believe in his supernatural powers and in his ability to deal with the unseen, mysterious forces of health and disease. The shaman draws upon the image of mystic authority that his culture places upon his profession. . . . The tension and stress created in the patient's mind by his illness can be neutralized immediately by the awesome position of the shaman as a supporting personality with superhuman forces at his disposal. (p. 86)

34. Roeschemeyer, Doctors and lawyers.

Later it is clear that Rogers understands the psychic as opposed to the physical effect of shamanistic methods:

> The shaman's primary attack on the sickness of his patients is psychotherapeutic. . . . Many of his patients, for a variety of reasons, suffer directly or indirectly from emotional disturbance. . . . Shamanistic therapy involves various theoretical justifications and numerous ways of diverting or subverting the effects of an emotional disturbance. . . . We can appreciate that his methods, although often bizarre and peculiar to us, can often deal effectively with illness in ways analogous to those used by modern psychiatrists. (p. 132)

Psychiatrists might not be so pleased at his analogy and would see the shaman, as the holistic practitioner and (it must be admitted) the placebo-giver, as simply exercising and strengthening the bonds of transference, unless he also gives potions which might contain plant extracts of medicinal value.

As Rogers points out the dichotomy between body and soul so central to modern Western medical concepts and enshrined in the dictum of cellular pathology by Virchow that there are only diseases of cells has no place in shamanistic therapy. On the other hand it is hard to be sure that shamans conceive of disease as other than personalistic. They give holistic therapy, but they don't always have a logical concept of disease, even by their terms. The shaman has a large psychological role in treating patients through the "symbolism of his office and person," but he would not understand degenerative diseases or metabolic disorders. He might perceive bacterial disease as an alien invasion and certainly would understand emotional problems. Rogers emphasizes how important is the expectation of being healed for the success of the shaman's ministrations. Confident that he can help, the shaman transfers that confidence to the patient, and that self-confidence in itself must be helpful. Many physicians in Western society, on the other hand, having abandoned their paternalistic and authoritarian approaches, would feel embarrassed to suggest that their person can comfort their patients or, at least, that it should.

Summarizing the underlying therapeutic principles of shamanistic practice, Rogers emphasizes several features which are familiar to modern practitioners: (1) relaxation and reassurance is an important part of the shaman's technique and will have a familiar ring to readers and practitioners of "relaxation therapy"; (2) hypnotism is quite commonly used, along with suggestion, and this too has had a checkered career in western medical practice; (3) transference is as important for the shaman as it is for Western psychotherapists, and must account for at least some of what happens between shaman and patient;

(4) group support, not very much different from the groups to support many Western patients, also bring important therapeutic benefit; (5) catharsis brought about by reenactment of the crisis that gave rise to conflict will have a familiar ring to many, from psychoanalysts to drama therapists; (6) the feature that may be the most germane to placebo-giving is what Rogers calls "symbolic manipulation" during the rites. Much of the symbolism is esoteric, but some of it is known to the patients and the spectators and is "psychologically important as a part of the healing procedure. It gives the patient the feeling that the dread mystery of his illness is being combatted by the ancient mysteries of his culture, and that the shaman is a qualified and certified technician of these mysteries" (p. 143).

This brief review of the shaman's activity raises as many questions as answers. Rogers states that "the healing of illness in any culture involves four questions: What is the nature and name of the malady? What caused it? What should be done to treat it? What are the patient's possibilities of recovery?" (p. 163). Diagnosis, etiology, treatment and prognosis are the names by which these activities go in Western medicine. I can do no better, however, than to give Rogers's conclusions:

> The large body of data in the literature of ethnography, travel and exploration that touches upon the methods of the shaman should be regarded as more than a cabinet of curiosa. It can properly be considered a corpus of findings from the great laboratory of non-western man and culture. While not reported in the systems and syntax of western science, it nonetheless provides a summary of much human experience dealing with the mind and the body and the relationship between the two. These data can well be examined in order to determine what avenues in investigation may have promise of value for future research. (p. 173)

I should note in closing, however, that in this all too brief review of the shaman, I have ignored—as Rogers has ignored—any contribution of herbs and potions that the shaman or other healer in preliterate societies may use. The lessons of folk medicine and the contributions of native remedies to the pharmacopoeia are too well known to demean their possible contributions.

Acupuncture. In the West acupuncture is regarded as only (1) anesthesia for painless surgery, or (2) analgesia—relief of symptoms by the application of needles to set points in the skin.[35] For Eastern

35. Steiner, R. P., Acupuncture: Cultural perspectives, *Postgrad. Med. Columbia* 74:60–78, 1983.

practitioners acupuncture is much more: it relieves pain as part of a much wider world view of health and disease. Western physicians examine only its physiological effect to compare it to placebo intervention, as I have done. Yet to look at acupuncture as a part of traditional Chinese medicine provides another salutary parallel to Western medicine in this most developed of all non-Western naturalistic schemes with its 5,000-year-old tradition.

As Dianne Connelly has pointed out, acupuncture used as an adjunct of Western medicine as a kind of fix like aspirin for a headache misses "the complex of mind/body causes out of which symptoms derive."[36] Haley Seif, a Yale College student learning to be expert in acupuncture, wrote to me that "Chinese medicine is geared toward treating diseases that conventional medicine considers too nonspecific to treat. This is because Chinese medicine focuses on correcting minor imbalances before they become acute. Examples of such conditions are a low energy, headaches, cold limbs, anxiety."[37] Such disorders, of course, are the same kinds of symptoms that the Western practitioner is likely to call "functional," and treat with tranquilizers or placebos. She continues, "Chinese medicine has also been quite successful in treating chronic disorders like hypertension, arthritis, asthma." These are disorders which Western practitioners treat with drugs, although in their minor forms they are likely to respond to any form of therapy or support. (I would add peptic ulcer to that list, as the controlled clinical trials discussed in chapter 2 have suggested.) But the point is that the nature of the therapy makes very little difference to the 80 percent of patients whose illnesses—or better, whose complaints—will disappear on their own or will respond to many different kinds of support.

Chinese physicians, Seif points out, "are shocked by the fact that many US medications have only been in use since the 1960s and the long term consequences of consuming these very strong chemical substances are not clear." The rejoinder that herbal medicines contain extracts that have sometimes proven harmful to patients suggests that reevaluation of both positions is in order. There must be some truth to what a Chinese folk practitioner said to Seif: "There should be a law that says people should not start medications for high blood pressure until they have tried some form of alternative medical treatment."

As I have emphasized elsewhere, a prominent specialist in hypertension said to me that a third of the patients in his clinic could stop taking their medications and remain healthy, but the task of survey-

36. Connelly, D. M., *Traditional acupuncture*, Columbia, Md.: Centre for Traditional Acupuncture, 1975.
37. Seif, H., personal communication, 1983.

ing them for complications or for the return of hypertension seemed so great and the anxiety they might feel at getting no medication, made him and his colleagues decide that giving medication was the easiest solution. Clearly their patients are taking impure placebos.

Acupuncture is part of a naturalistic system developed over five thousand years ago. Connelly suggests that a basic difference between Western and Eastern thought is that in the West, "We have philosophical traditions and cultures that emphasize the concept of 'either/or', forcing us to continually make comparisons, choices, and judgements of one thing over another." For the Eastern tradition, on the other hand, "the concepts of 'both/and', . . . [represent] the underlying philosophy, two concepts which are never realities, each present in the other, both present in the whole."

The so-called *Ch'i* (vital life force) provides the basic philosophy for Chinese medicine. It holds that acupuncture works via pathways of energy called *meridians*. These are visible to experts as small spots close to the surface of the skin which represent the acupuncture points, stimulation of which influences the energy of the body. Diagnostic techniques include observation, the sense of smell, listening, touch ("the 12 pulses") and much more: The ideal practitioner of Chinese medicine looks at the whole person: "Also integrated are colors, dreams, family and social relations, self-expression, love, spirituality, and the belief that not all can be explained and dissected."

Connelly points out that

> the concept of balance that I have referred to is perhaps the most powerful perspective that acupuncture has to offer. Central to it is the requirement that the individual human in pain must be an active agent in the process of re-balancing, not "done to" by a professional, but informed and mobilized throughout. . . . The patient must be seen and experienced as a whole—not as a collection of symptoms or even imbalances or blockages.

Chinese medicine can be regarded as logical, traditional, holistic, and internally consistent as long as the tests of the Western biomedical scientist are not applied. Like all other naturalistic schemes, it has lessons for us not necessarily in its specifics, but in making physicians recognize that the medical system is a cultural system with its own concepts, theories, practices, and agreed-upon ways of looking at matters. Western practitioners should not adopt the theories of Chinese practitioners, but they should look at their successes and the successes of the indigenous practitioners regardless of the culture to learn to be skeptical about native medicines and also about what we do.

Paul Wolpe, whose comments on Chinese acupuncture and on

Western medicine's cooptation of it, have been most helpful to me, wrote:

> Why shouldn't Western practitioners take a serious look at Chinese *therapeutics?* It is, in my opinion, ultimately anthropocentric to suppose that a 5,000-year-old tradition, developed by what was until the eighteenth century undoubtedly the most scientifically advanced culture on earth, is no more than placebo. The Chinese culture is too sophisticated to rest on ineffective therapeutics. Let us suppose for just one moment that chi exists, and that the Chinese theory of etiology—that disease starts long before its manifestation in symptoms through the weakening of a bodily subsystem—is correct. If disease can be prevented, or morbidity reduced, by balancing energy flows, that should be empirically verifiable. Doesn't it make more sense to research it than to dismiss it all as placebo?[38]

Hwa-Byung. Hwa-Byung offers an exotic example of how culture influences the choice of symptoms.[39] Among the Chinese and Koreans somaticization has been a common acceptable outlet for stress. The Chinese man who has too many troubles will not complain, "I am under too much pressure," but rather, "I have a headache or a stomach ache" as his way of complaining about the stress. (Whether the Western metaphor of "pressure" is a better one is a subject all in itself.) The system of Chinese medicine is characterized by an organ-oriented concept of pathology, so much so that many Chinese patients are reluctant to express emotions except as somatic complaints. In Chinese society somatic illness is an "effective and legitimate excuse to request rest and care from others, while psychological strain is not. . . . Thus, patients learn how to present their problems in terms of somatic complaints to give a signalled illness effectively."[40] Obviously so ready an acceptance of somatic illness with so little acceptance of psychiatric problems makes people reluctant to explore their emotional problems. As their culture reinforces hypochondriasis, Tseng points out, many Chinese people will find bodily sensations a convenient scapegoat.

With this background, the clinician who reads of Hwa-Byung, a syndrome common among Koreans, will recognize a familiar "depres-

38. Wolpe, P. R., The maintenance of professional authority: Acupuncture and the American physician, *Social Problems* 32:409–24, 1985.

39. Lin, K. M., Hwa-Byung: A Korean cultural syndrome? *Amer. J. Psychiatr.* 140: 105–07, 1983.

40. Tseng, W. S., The nature of somatic complaints among psychiatric patients: The Chinese case, *Comp. Psychiatry* 16:237–45, 1945.

sive equivalent" rather than anything exotic.[41] Patients with Hwa-Byung complain of indigestion, anorexia, dyspnea, palpitation, generalized aches, and the sensation of a mass in the epigastrium. Upon analysis such patients turn out to be depressed and, in the only English-language report, its psychological origin is underlined. To the American practitioner the conviction that a mass is present will be strange, but the rest will be familiar.

Abdominal pain. We need not turn far for other examples of how culture defines disease. A forty-five-year-old American woman with lower abdominal pain and an unfaithful husband may, depending upon her views of life, see a clergyman, a lawyer, or any of an array of physicians. The lawyer may see his task as arranging a divorce—for which he gets paid—or a reconciliation; the clergyman may strive to keep the marriage together, or may act as a therapist, or both. If the woman chooses a physician, the gastroenterologist, gynecologist, or urologist will each invade quite different orifices to offer different interpretations of what is wrong.

Even today different social classes in America and Britain may give different descriptions of the same sensations. The more educated and sophisticated may talk of "stress," while the uneducated are freer to talk of "pain," where once they might have talked of lizards.

The lizard in the stomach. A lizard in the stomach figures prominently in Cabot's discussion of lying to patients and much is made of the bizarre quality of the complaint. Lizards, it turns out, however, can get into the stomach by personalistic or naturalistic routes: "A recurring theme in witchcraft belief is that animals are present in the body, introduced by magical means."[42] In view of Richard Cabot's comments on the woman who complained that she had a lizard in her stomach (see chapter 9) and in view of the unattributed comments of Freud on this same matter, it is interesting to note that Snow finds "animal intrusion" as a cause of illness to have a long history in European and American folklore. "Spring lizards" as well as other animals can grow in the stomach from drinking river water that contains eggs, according to folklore. Fear of having a lizard in the stomach is not then quite as unnatural as Cabot and other physicians reading his account apparently believed. But we do not know the ethnic or national origins of Cabot's patient.

Other physicians might have failed to rout the "lizard" because they did not possess "special powers" to keep other lizards from growing in the stomach; their failure might have had nothing to do

41. Lin, Hwa-Byung.
42. Snow, Folk medical beliefs.

with their lying about therapy. In the black culture described by Snow, healing is seen as a gift from God, a gift more important than any training. Where a relatively coherent set of beliefs exists, placebo would be no more likely to help than any other agents introduced by a nonblessed practitioner.

Diseases of civilization. Of course, some disorders could not exist without certain cultural artifacts. In a society without telephones disturbed people could not annoy others with phone calls. In a medieval society without clocks Type A behavior must have been improbable. Anorexia nervosa, a disease of rich and plenty, might go unrecognized in an area of famine. Indeed the young woman with anorexia nervosa in such circumstances might be seen as a heroine because of her apparent fortitude and hyperactivity. In our affluent society, as Fabrega suggests, wrinkles can come to seem a legitimate concern, a "disease" almost, and facelifts a triumph of medical skills.[43] Other such examples will come to mind.

Criticisms of Anthropological Studies

Spontaneous recovery. Most patients get better and most complaints run their course and go away, in primitive as well as in civilized life. It is easy then to mistake an intervention for effective when it has simply come at the right time to take credit. That is as true of Western medical practices as of primitive cures.

Lieban points out that

perception of medical realities can be obfuscated by a number of factors in situations where modern medicine is effective and/or indigenous medicine is not.

1. Most illnesses eventually end in spontaneous recovery. When this occurs and the patients have been treated by local healers, confidence in indigenous medicine may be bolstered by cures for which it is only fortuitously connected.

2. When therapy for an illness is sought from both a physician and a healer, the physician may cure the patient and the healer get the credit.

3. Purposes as well as results of modern medicine may be misperceived.[44]

Confusion between illness and disease. Anthropologists and sociologists alike rightfully criticize physicians for paying little attention to

43. Fabrega, The need for an ethnomedical science.
44. Lieban, R., The field of medical anthropology, in Landy, *Culture, disease, and healing*, pp. 13–31.

the cultural meaning of disease. Anthropologists, on the other hand, can be faulted for paying almost no attention to the distinctions between illness and disease, between complaints of pain and organic processes. If 80 percent of illnesses in modern Western society are the result of stress or culture, or are self-limited, then any intervention may prove useful, but we should not ascribe to shamans or other healers more than can be proven.

As I suggested earlier, the major obstacle for the physician surveying medical anthropology lies in the unsophisticated acceptance by the anthropologist of all complaints as "diseases." While modern medicine has focused too much on the specific biological cause of diseases and not enough on the economic, social, political, or cultural factors which account for so much human illness,[45] anthropologists seem to regard all testimony about clinical improvement as more or less to be accepted. Discussions of shamans offer considerable analysis of the concept and role of the shaman, how people become shamans, and how they go about their work, but really very little about the kinds of disorders or complaints that they treat. Anthropologists need more active collaboration from trained physicians to separate pain and suffering, which clearly can be relieved, from the cure of disease.

Because medical anthropologists do not distinguish between illness and disease, they make comments such as the following: "Only fringe practitioners in western countries hope to use the theories of the Five Elements, of yin and yang, or the meridians. These theories belong in the domain of historians and cultural anthropologists. . . . Although useful medications have been derived from the traditional Asian pharmacopoeias, few new discoveries are likely to come from this direction."[46] Set that comment against Seif: "Chinese medicine has slowly and carefully developed techniques to discover imbalances before they manifest in an overtly physical way in the body. . . . Chinese medicine is geared toward treating diseases that conventional medicine considers too non-specific to treat."[47] Or the following from Lock's book on East Asian medicine: "All diseases can be thought of as energy problems," states Dr. Nagai; "They can be detected through pulse diagnosis long before changes are visible microscopically." He adds that "by the time a disease is developed to a secondary, visible state, it is sometimes already too late to stop it. If a potential disease is caught very early, then precise analysis is not necessary: although the form of a future disease is not yet manifest."[48]

Clearly the Western anthropologist Leslie is concerned only with

45. Cassell, *The healer's art.*
46. Leslie, quoted in Landy, *Culture, disease, and healing,* p. 511.
47. Seif, personal communication.
48. Lock, M., *East Asian medicine in urban Japan,* Berkeley: University of California Press, 1980.

diseases, although he appears too skeptical of empiric therapy and what can be learned from it. Lock and Seif are clearly enthusiasts, but they are talking about illnesses, complaints, or symptoms that make up that 80 percent of problems that the placebo helps. Controlled trials to establish the accuracy of such assertions about "predisease" are in order.

The distress or disorders which are relieved by native healers seem to an outside observer to be either self-limited disorders or disorders of functional or emotional origin. Even the reports most deferred to inescapably describe functional disorders. For example, Pattison, a psychiatrist, in an otherwise very thoughtful essay, describes a young Indian girl diagnosed as having "acute schizophrenia" who was cured of her delusions by exorcism.[49] Kleinman discusses several cases in an interesting paper, but the symptoms relieved or explained are those which most clinicians would see as stemming from depression or hostility or representing withdrawn behavior, and the like.[50]

It may not go far enough to say that only emotional or functional disorders are relieved by faith or by healers in preliterate societies. Yet it seems likely that the special kinds of relief evoked by primitive healers have largely to do with pain and suffering, distress, impotence, musculoskeletal disorders, and such. There may be exceptions, but the reports that I have read describe the same self-limited events or functional disorders which comprise so much of a Western physician's office practice. Only rarely is intractable or serious disease described. For example, in their study of rural medicine in Greece, symptoms that Blum and Blum report as the "effects of the evil eye" that yield to healers include headaches, dizziness, sleeplessness, weakness, fretfulness, numbness, yawning, and vomiting.[51] These are complaints that most physicians would recognize as coming from tension and yielding to any charismatic approach.

The tang-ki. Kleinman, studying indigenous practitioners in Taiwan, emphasizes that the *tang-ki* treated what Westerners would largely call psychosomatic and emotional disorders:

As we have seen, indigenous practitioners primarily treat three types of disorders: 1) acute, self-limited (naturally remitting) diseases; 2) non-life threatening, chronic diseases in which manage-

49. Pattison, E., Psychosocial interpretation of exorcism, *J. Operational Psychiatry* 8:5–21, 1977.

50. Kleinman, A., Neurasthenia and depression, *Culture, Medicine, and Psychiatry* 6:117–90, 1982; Kleinman, A. and Sung, L., Why do indigenous practitioners successfully heal? *Social Science and Medicine* 13B:7–26, 1976.

51. Blum, R., and Blum, B., *Health and healing in rural Greece*, Stanford: Stanford University Press, 1965.

ment of illness (psychosocial and cultural) problems is a larger component of clinical management than biomedical treatment of the disease; and 3) secondary somatic manifestations (somatization) of minor psychological disorders and interpersonal problems. The treatment of disease plays a small role in the care of these disorders.[52]

Taiwanese patients go to a Western-style physician for biologically originating diseases but choose their indigenous healers for "the treatment of fright." Surprisingly enough, Kleinman suggests that indigenous therapy may be effective against diseases, as well as illnesses, by exerting "placebo or direct effect upon such diseases." He displays more faith in placebo therapy than in the ministrations of the tang-ki.

In an extraordinarily illuminating view of how healers work in the context of a culture, Kleinman reemphasizes how the modern Western "professional practitioner is trained to ignore illness systematically as part of his exclusive interest in the recognition and treatment of disease. He is taught to cure, not to care. This profound distortion of clinical work is built into the biomedical training of physicians."[53]

The more I read, however, of anthropological studies of disease, the more I am troubled by their ready acceptance of folk healing, cult healing, and all the rest. There needs to be a more vigorous comparison of the outcome of diseases looked at by medical anthropologists; it needs to be as rigorous as the studies by medical practitioners of the outcome of disease. "Lastly, only by addressing clinically relevant questions from its unique perspective can medical anthropology exert a practical effect on the practice and teaching of clinical medicine and psychiatry."[54]

Biomedical model and medical anthropology. Although Kleinman believes that the biomedical model is not the only one by which medical anthropologists should judge healing, and although he hopes to protect medical anthropology "from the increasing if usually disguised reliance on biomedical presuppositions and categories,"[55] it is not clear why it is necessary to avoid the biomedical model. It is important not to rely on it exclusively is what I think he means. Indeed, given the success of that model in the treatment and analysis of biological phenomena in human disease, as long as we keep in mind the distinctions, it would be confusing to equate relief of complaints with cure of disease.

52. Kleinman, A., *Patients and healers in the context of culture*, Berkeley: University of California Press, 1980, p. 361.
53. Ibid., p. 376.
54. Ibid., p. 363.
55. Ibid., p. 378.

Looking at nonbiomedical approaches to pain and suffering helps the Western health professional to begin to try to order his own way of thinking about such matters. After all the Western health professional, physician, nurse, or nurse practitioner is trained to deal with disease in a specific, logical, and rational way. He can be open to other forms of therapy without abandoning his fundamental training and logical approach. The faith healer or folk practitioner, on the other hand, has no background in rational medicine and cannot cross the barrier to examine and utilize technical scientific approaches. But considerations of these somewhat arcane issues may help Western practitioners grasp what kinds of diseases or complaints could be handled outside the usual medical context. There might even be some economic incentive to do so, as the costs of medical technology grow and as the money to pay for tests shrinks. It is not easy to get either doctor or patient to recognize that not every complaint deserves a work-up and a specific diagnosis. If symptoms are relieved, we can defer the full diagnostic barrage.

Mechanisms of folk healing. Mechanisms postulated for most successful folk healing seem to be largely "psychosomatic" and no different from those proposed for the placebo discussed in chapter 12. The hypothalamus, endorphins, or control of the immunological system by the brain are all cited. The metaphor of the machine is invoked, to talk of the autonomic nervous system being "tuned up" or "unbalanced." The psychoanalysts consider the symbolic effect of such manipulations (or placebos) and find the ability of the patient to trust or to become dependent an important feature. Most explanations so far seem more theory than observation, but are valuable as hypothesis generation, as long as they are not accepted prematurely without evidence.

PSYCHOSOMATIC MEDICINE

When doctors call a disease *psychosomatic*, they usually mean that it is a disease which is either (1) caused by emotional factors or (2) made worse by emotional factors. For the former *psychogenic* would be a more appropriate term. To say that a disease is made worse by the emotions takes into account the multifactorial origin of most diseases and what goes into making an illness. That latter use is the more appropriate, but to say that something is psychosomatic is often to suggest that it is caused by the mind, something that very few physicians currently believe. In general, therefore, the term has fallen in esteem in the 1980s, but *psychosomatic* might be salvaged if it could be redefined to refer to illness and to include cultural as well as psychic and biological influences. Psychosomatic medicine, however defined, is clearly an important consideration in thinking about the placebo.

In general the original narrow definition was a good one: psychosomatic medicine was the study of "the interrelationships between emotional life and bodily processes both normal and pathologic."[56] Today we would add "and of the mind," partly because Cartesian dualism seems unattractive in a time when we know that a neurotransmitter such as cholecystokinin, a hormone found originally in the gut, is also present in the brain and is probably ubiquitous as a neurotransmitter. What psychosomatic medicine is *not* is a belief that diseases are caused *only* by the mind and emotions. The term implies, or should imply, the conviction that *no* disease is free of emotional aspects, or—in the terms that I have been using in this book—no disease is without its accompanying illness, in every conscious person.

Psychosomatic medicine, in a sense, looks at disease from the far end of the telescope, seeing it in the context of life. Unlike the reductionist the physician sensitive to psychosomatic issues sees the patient as the proverbial person. There can be no clear separation of the psychosomatic from the other parts of medicine. For example, psychiatry has for its domain diseases which are at least functionally "of the mind," but discoveries of the past decade suggest that even mental states may have a biochemical locus. The reductionist will bring all disease to molecules and will agree with the modern biochemically oriented psychiatrist. But we clinicians have to deal with people and in our daily activities we can function quite well with such rough categories as medicine, psychosomatic, and psychiatry. After all, the gastroenterologist and cardiologist roughly divide up their terrains without worrying too much about the borders.

In the 1940s psychosomatic medicine flourished as leaders like Franz Alexander and Flanders Dunbar barraged the willing student with the idea that specific emotions led to specific diseases.[57] Whether theorists of that time thought that specific personality types were associated with specific disorders, and who was responsible for the "specificity" hypotheses, are issues less important today than the overall if distant influence of the movement. Bringing back to prominence ideas of mind/body relationships which had lain dormant since the advent of cellular pathology was no mean achievement.[58] Ackerknecht suggests that psychosomatic medicine as a theory and practice

56. Editors, Introductory statement, *Psychosom. Med.* 1:3–5, 1939.
57. Alexander, F., *Psychosomatic medicine.* New York: Norton, 1950; Dunbar, F., *Emotions and bodily changes,* 4th ed., New York: Columbia University Press, 1954.
58. Lipowski, Z. J., What does the word "psychosomatic" really mean? A historical and semantic inquiry, *Psychosomatic Med.* 46:153–71, 1984.

is far older, however, and that it can be traced to the Greeks. Hippocratic medicine was largely somatic, avoiding the mystical and magical Aesculapian medicine of the Greek temples that Edelstein has described so well.[59] For the Hippocratic practitioners treatment of the soul or the psyche was to be avoided. Yet Ackerknecht reminds us of Plato's remarks on the helpfulness of "fair words" for the soul and suspects that the Aesculapians had a long-lasting influence.[60] Ackerknecht emphasizes how the "passions" for the ensuing two thousand years have been deemed important for medical practice: Galen directed attention to the role of the emotions in pathogenesis and treatment with the goal of freeing man from his "passions." Those who think, for example, that Norman Cousins had a new idea in healing with laughter will be surprised to learn that Maimonides recommended the stimulation of psychic energies through "perfumes, music and enjoyable stories." In modern times William Beaumont showed how the emotions influenced gastric secretion in his voyageur St. Martin.

The details of such experiments are fascinating but of less importance to us at the moment except to remind us that the tradition has been a long one. The modern psychosomatic movement may not have recognized its roots in the past, but its influence for good and bad is still with us. Alexander emphasized the "logic of the emotions," the affinity of specific emotional factors for specific aspects of the autonomic nervous system. His was, as Powell has pointed out, a dynamically oriented etiologic system.[61] On the other hand the more religious philosophical background of Flanders Dunbar made her look at the person as a whole in a more interventional therapeutic approach.

The psychosomatic movement may have erred in emphasizing the idea that a specific personality or a specific way of reacting to an emotion brought about a specific disease. It foundered on the notion probably fostered by those outside the movement, that the psyche caused disease, and in part could not resolve the mind-brain dilemma. That is certainly not what Alexander explicitly wrote, and the characterization may have been an unfair one by those unreceptive to such ideas. Yet Jung's comments encapsulate a view. "A discovery which is very unwelcome to the science of medicine: namely, the discovery that the psyche is an aetiological or causal factor in disease. In the course

59. Edelstein, L., The professional ethics of the Greek physician, *Bull. Hist. Med.* 30:391–419, 1956.

60. Ibid., and Ackerknecht, E. H., The notion of psychosomatic medicine, *Psychological Med.* 12:17–24, 1982.

61. Powell, R. C., Helen Flanders Dunbar (1902–1959) and a holistic approach to psychosomatic problems. I. The rise and fall of a medical philosophy, *Psychiatric Quarterly* 49:133–52, 1977.

of the nineteenth century medicine shaped its methods and theory in such a way as to become one of the disciplines of natural science, and it also adopted that primary assumption of natural science: material causation."[62]

Present-day psychiatrists are trying to regain acceptance as neuro-biologists and welcome material causation. Specifically, I suspect, they welcome the biomedical idea that finding biochemical derangements in patients with mental disorders means that those aberrancies are the cause of the mental state.

Still, the conviction that a person is part of his culture and that embedded in his physiology lie reactions to specific situations is an important one which has been revived as "holistic medicine." The approach was dogmatic to be sure and Mack Lipkin has emphasized to me how Franz Alexander with his commanding stature, impressive Berlin accent, and immense self-confidence dominated the field.[63] So compelling was his personality and that of Dunbar that their followers saw only what these leaders wanted them to see. "Holistic medicine" lacks the outstanding personality of a Dunbar or Alexander.

Margaret Mead stressed the importance of looking at the culture and society of the sick person. In a paper which deserves rereading, "The Concept of Culture and the Psychosomatic Approach," she said: "That at the functioning of every part of the human body is moulded by the culture within which the individual has been reared. . . . Also by the way that he, born into a society with a definite culture, has been fed and disciplined, fondled and put to sleep, punished and rewarded."[64] Holistic medical practitioners would have little quarrel with Margaret Mead:

> The disease must have been seen as systematically related to the total mode of behaviour of the patient, to his total personality. The student of psychosomatic medicine was saying that in order to understand the pattern of psychodynamics, we had to go to the life history of the individual patient. . . .
>
> The cultural pattern is built into his whole personality in one process in which no dualism exists so that the temper tantrum, the tautened muscles, the change in the manufacturing of blood sugar, and the verbal insults hurled at an offending parent, all become patterned and integrated. . . .
>
> The psychosomatic theorist will have made a considerable ad-

62. Jung, C., *Modern man in search of a soul*, New York: Harcourt, Brace, Jovanovich, 1933, p. 222.

63. Lipkin, M., personal communication, 1984.

64. Mead, M., Concept of culture and the psychosomatic approach, *Psychiatry* 10:57–76, 1947.

vance in the invocation of culture in his thinking if he can think of two individuals from different cultural backgrounds, as he might think of the manifestations of Reynaud's disease under different temperature conditions.

In the 1930s and 1940s interest in nutrition was almost as avid as it is today, fostered then by the recent discovery of vitamins and emphasis on constituents of the diet. The likening of culture to diet finds a familiar metaphorical echo today, when nutrition and interest in high-fiber diets have been so renewed. "The culture may be likened to the standard diet in which the individual members have subsisted since birth." Psychosomatic considerations would caution those who ascribe changes in gastrointestinal diseases simply to changes in diet, for example, and not to a change in culture, to have some reservations about recommending fundamental changes in the American diet and not in its psyche.

The relationship of psychosomatic medicine to holistic medicine needs consideration. The practitioners of holistic medicine seized upon a notion without analysis and have taken all observations as the equal of each others. I do not know whether the systems-approach is needed or whether a less intellectual approach will do. Psychosomatic medicine teaches us that a person is born into a culture, and that his physiological systems and ways of reacting are as influenced by individual experiences with his parents, his surroundings, and his culture as is his language. I like the definition of the psychosomaticist as the physician who specializes in listening,[65] but psychosomatics could be so much more.

Acupuncture

One form of alternative medicine that makes little claim beyond relief of pain is acupuncture, at least as it has permeated research institutions; in the West its origin in a wider worldview has been submerged by the dramatic benefit of analgesia. I intend here to review only some parallels with the placebo. That acupuncture needling of specific points in the body remote from where the patient feels pain may relieve that pain seems to be agreed. What is not known is how often pain is relieved, whether the benefit is more than that of a placebo, whether the relief is adequately explained by the theory behind acupuncture, and whether the results are predictable—and repeatable. I cannot tell from my reading whether acupuncture needling stimulates endogenous opioids or not. I suspect that it does, but current evidence is not sufficiently convincing to let me decide whether

65. Lipowski, What does the word "psychosomatic" really mean, and Lipowski, Z. J., Psychosocial aspects of disease, *Ann. Intern. Med.* 71:1197–1206, 1969.

placebos or acupuncture stimulate endorphins in the blood or spinal fluid and to what degree.

Mechanisms and effectiveness. We have to ask (1) Does acupuncture work? (2) On whom does it work? (3) How does it work? (4) How often does it work? Then, assessing it as we would any new approach, we should compare it to other forms of therapy in acute and chronic disorders and, finally, ascertain whether acupuncture improves the long-term outlook for some pain patients. The quite contentious varying views lead to the conclusion that nobody has the answers. Reviews in 1985 suggest that acupuncture relieves pain overall in about 60 percent of the patients at a rate, I think, not so much different from placebos. The relief of pain by acupuncture is sometimes very quick, almost immediate, but sometimes relief is very slow. The duration of relief is unpredictable.

As a clinician I have some concern about reported clinical studies. A report from Texas is typical.[66] That paper claimed to show that acupuncture relieved the "chronic pain syndrome" in twenty patients because it raised their metenkephalin levels. The authors reported that clinical relief of pain was accompanied by lessening of accompanying psychiatric symptoms. Nevertheless, reading the methods, I find that the only pain accepted for treatment was that which was *not* caused by "an identifiable, currently active surgical and/or medical condition." I was surprised to find that patients with such chronic pain were able to tolerate being taken off *all* medication for at least ten days before they started acupuncture therapy. We are not told how they were feeling during that preliminary vigil—whether they were free of pain. Nor do the authors tell us whether their patients could go about their usual activities or whether their pain was so heightened by omitting their usual drugs that *any* therapy might have helped. A skeptical reader is left with a feeling that patients who could bear pain for at least ten days before taking on acupuncture therapy might not have needed any kind of therapy. Further, the patients, to quote the authors, "were also experiencing serious psychiatric difficulties." In the absence of a control or a "placebo" group it is hard to remain convinced by any reported improvement. Further studies may well prove that endorphins are stimulated by acupuncture and that pain is relieved by mechanisms specific to acupuncture, but evidence so far brings little conviction.

One of the leading proponents of acupuncture in Great Britain,

66. Kiser, R. S., Gatchel, R. J., Bhatia, K., et al., Acupuncture relief of chronic pain syndrome correlates with increased plasma met-enkephalin concentration, *Lancet* 2:1394–96, 1983.

George Lewith, agrees that controls using physical placebos are needed to prove the benefit of acupuncture.[67] He accepts, however, only a 30 percent relief rate as opposed to the claimed 60 percent relief rate for acupuncture, admitting even so that it is not going to be easy to prove the benefits of acupuncture by such trials. Elsewhere in Great Britain placebo studies of duodenal ulcer pain show that placebos bring only a 30 percent relief in Britain, in contrast to the 60 percent relief in the United States. I cannot place very much confidence then in the arithmetic differences between 30 percent and 60 percent. Mendelson,[68] who has conducted controlled trials of acupuncture, states, "The placebo component is clinically more important than its physiological effects."[69]

I conclude that because there are so many different kinds of pain, experimental and clinical, so many different expectations from such different patients that satisfying studies of the mechanism of acupuncture will be long awaited. How much benefit comes from the person doing the procedure and how much comes from the process is uncertain, but the same criticism is leveled at psychotherapy, placebo, and other forms of intervention. How much is specific to the technique and how much just a consequence of sustained effort, attention, transference, and hope I do not know. Such comments do not denigrate the need for further study, nor intend that acupuncture has no place, but emphasize the importance of the rational, reasonable gathering of data. If in the end acupuncture turns out to be only a placebo, as I suspect it may, then it still may be a powerful tool with a specific, predictable, useful place in therapy—if enough observations are made.

HOLISTIC MEDICINE / ALTERNATIVE MEDICINE

In the process of reflecting on these matters, I wondered whether the holistic movement has the right idea. In many ways some of the ideals of some proponents of holism are on target, to heal the conceptual split of body and mind in medicine, the bequest of Cartesian dualism. If that was the major aim, there would be little problem for me. But I found a disappointing, almost indefinable collection of theories and practice, encompassing so wide a variety of approaches that almost no discussion can encompass them. Some of the more reason-

67. Lewith, G. T., and Machin, D., On the evaluation of the clinical effects of acupuncture, *Pain* 16:111–27, 1983.

68. Mendelson, G., Acupuncture, *Brit. Med. J.* 288:1999, 1984.

69. Mendelson, G., Selwood, T. S., Kranz, H., et al., Acupuncture treatment of chronic low back pain, *Amer. J. Med.* 74:49–55, 1983.

able approaches simply offer a comprehensive person-oriented medical care, but others come close to quackery: "Well-intentioned 'healers' may adopt this label (holism) to gain acceptance for methods that after scientific investigation may prove to have little or no benefit. Charlatans may exploit the term 'holistic health' in promoting their useless remedies."[70]

There has been no firm definition of holistic medicine. The very term *holistic* has become so contaminated that I doubt that it can be rehabilitated. *Holistic* has it origin in a book, *Holism and Evolution*, written, surprisingly enough, by the late South African Prime Minister and World War II leader, Jan Christian Smuts. He took the word *holism* from the Greek *holos* meaning "whole." Smuts's book is said to be an indictment of reductionism.

It is difficult to generalize about holistic practitioners. Fitzgerald divides some of the "more scandalous" practitioners of alternative medicine into: (1) the true believers, for whom concepts of health and disease are a true religion, "on a different plane of thought" from others; 2) the mercantilists, quacks no more than con artists for whom a "secret remedy" provides a way to make a living.[71] She blames their success on the gullibility of the American public, as uncritical of science as of scam. She questions whether it is prudent, financially at least, for scientists to have to disprove every "crazy idea."

Lisa Newton takes the holistic health movement to be primarily a "social movement" made up as much of self-healers as of physicians.[72] In many ways she is right to make us think of holistic medicine in that way, more like a mob than a unified, coherent movement. Everybody in the current movement goes his own way defining disease and cure any way he wants, usually taking a part for the whole. Massage is good for aches and pains (as we have seen, possibly by stimulating the gate mechanism), and doubtless also overcomes loneliness, but it should not be elevated to a "method" of healing. Looking into the eyes is helpful to practitioner and poet alike, but iridology claims to discern all diseases by looking at the iris. Many other pretentious claims are made. Even the "Holistic Medical Association" looks to an outsider like a group huddled together against attack rather than having a firm body of knowledge and practice on which most of its members agree. Made up of D.O. and M.D. physicians, the association accepts medication and even surgery as therapeutic "modalities,"

70. Kopelman, L., and Moskop, J., The holistic health movement: A survey and critique, *J. Med. Philosph.* 6:209–35, 1981.

71. Fitzgerald, F. T., Science and Scam: Alternative thought patterns in alternative health care, *NEJM* 309:1066–67, 1983.

72. Newton, L., personal communication, 1985.

and does not repudiate conventional medicine—but that is about as far as agreement goes.

By and large adherents to holistic health movements share certain characteristics, some specifically directed at ways of keeping healthy through daily habits, ways of eating, and what used to be called "physical culture." Others, more theoretical, provide a philosophical outlook that permeates the practices associated with holism.

Self-care plays the largest role; this involves spiritual, mental, and environmental concerns as well as more purely physical ones. Even when the holistic practitioner is a physician, the holistic health medicine movement would make the patient as responsible for his "health" as the physician. People in the holistic movement are urged to keep physically fit, to learn how to cope with stress, and to eat food which is believed to be healthy, avoiding products considered harmful. (In the holistic movement, the gastroenterologist father convinced of the virtues of the high-fiber diet to prevent diseases of the gut can dine with his holistic vegetarian child in one great, if gassy, festival of love.)

There is a *distrust* of, even a distaste for, orthodox medical practices, which culminates in a particularly Luddite distrust of medical technology. Qualms about physicians and their instruments, along with a general skepticism about professionals generally, loom large in the holistic movement; even to one sympathetic to some of their goals, holistic enthusiasts seem to question traditional medical practices from too strong an adversarial standpoint. The People's Medical Society, for example, asks physicians to sign a pledge, the "Code of Practice" that almost presupposes that physicians are not to be trusted. On the other hand the holistic health movement takes on a paradoxically antiquarian air when it reverts to old traditions such as homeopathy that have been assimilated or discarded in modern medicine.

Holistic practitioners recognize that not all symptoms have an organic basis, but that many complaints arise from an emotional, cultural, and economic basis. Much emphasis is placed on enlarging and enhancing spiritual life. Finally, there is concern for the environment, not so much as a place of beauty and refuge as a potentially hostile origin of disease. By environment people in the holistic movement mean not only air and water, but our homes and society.

For a first-hand view, let us look at how a proponent of holistic medicine, himself a medical physician, defines the movement. The holistic practitioner, according to James S. Gordon,[73] (1) "sees the patient as a whole person"; (2) "views illness not as the enemy, but as a message and opportunity for inner growth"; (3) "feels that physicians

73. Gordon, J. S., quoted in M. L. Fuerst, Holistic Medicine, *Med. World News.* 25 July 1985, pp. 34–53.

can affect patients just by interacting with them"; (4) believes that "patients achieve health more easily when they collaborate with physicians than when they are simply told what to do." All in all these four tenets are certainly what this book has been all about, except for the idea that disease or illness should be looked at as a "welcome opportunity." Human beings have to accept diseases, too often, and to come to terms with them. But for most the notion that "you will be a better person afterward" is an achievement better avoided than gloried in. Disease is a misfortune to be faced and treated when possible for most of us, but it is accepted as a challenge for personal growth only by the most spiritual among us.

Still, it is only in the next two attitudes, as Dr. Gordon puts them, that some physicians would take issue. "Physicians don't treat patients as much as teach them how to remain healthy." He should have added *try to* remain healthy. Smoking cigarettes has proven harmful, along with being too fat or drinking too much alcohol, or not getting any exercise at all. Yet all of us envy those people who drink, eat, and smoke too much even at the funerals of their more abstemious friends. Their genes have something to do with their good fortune and their good luck reminds us that we may be able to keep from harming ourselves, but that remaining healthy is beyond our current accomplishments. Doctors, like Galston's Royal Family, do not live longer than other people. As I contemplate the legion of joggers rushing by with pained expressions, I wonder whether they are running away from something or running for something. Doctors can teach prudence, good public and personal hygiene, we can even council against destroying health, but really cannot do much, so far, about teaching people how to remain healthy. Reassessing, and changing, our lifestyles and priorities may be an important reaction to disease or illness, but physicians for the most part can act only as catalysts.

Such skepticism does not accord with the conclusions of the panels of eminent physicians often blessed by the Federal Government. Yet anyone watching the pendulum swings of what is acceptable and admirable must have doubts about the enthusiastically global assumptions of public health experts and holistic leaders alike.

Health is also defined rather exuberantly by the World Health Organization as "complete physical, mental, and social well-being and not merely the absence of disease or infirmity." Until we have gotten rid of disease and infirmity, doctors will do well to concentrate on their patients' diseases and illnesses.

Encouraging self-reliance is one of the more laudable qualities of holism. I see many patients who have become passive recipients of medical care, vessels waiting to be filled with drugs. I often wish— and usually tell them—that they must be active participants in their own return to health. "The doctors don't seem to be doing much for you. Why don't you try to do something more on your own?" The notion that the doctor does not treat disease is, to be charitable, a claim that Dr. Gordon must have made to be provocative.

Finally, Dr. Gordon states that holistic physicians have moved from "devotion to techniques of devotion." A wonderful turn of phrase even if his meaning eludes me. Devotion to God? To one's self? To exercise or meditation? Nor am I sure what is meant by "spirit" and what separates it from "mind." I do not know whether people who talk about "spirit" mean the soul, character, or if they know just exactly what they do mean. Yet despite the philosophical exhortation to define terms, I can live with the vaguely eschatological flavor that surrounds the term as some holistic practitioners use it.

From the foregoing I worry that holistic medicine, however praiseworthy its goals and however much I may agree with a lot of them, lacks a rational enough foundation and objective enough assessment to persuade me that, so far, it represents anything more than some well-intentioned physicians along with too many nonmedical enthusiasts for whom everything goes. The problem in holistic medicine lies not in its aims, but in the means by which they are achieved and the very spongy concepts described with wonderful words.

James talked of the "mind-cure movement" of the late nineteenth century. Its literature "is so moon-struck with optimism and so vaguely expressed that an academically trained intellect finds it almost impossible to read it at all."[74] Everything goes: if it feels good, it must be good for you. It is this unreasoning acceptance of almost any kind of approach that pains me. There is much to be hoped for, but much to be done.

The belief or, better, the faith of the person caught up in holistic health must contribute to his benefit, but whether this represents a placebo effect, I do not know. Later, however, I will comment on the relationship of groups to the "healing mode." There is certainly much good and usefulness in assuming personal responsibility and there certainly is no harm in many of the practices of holistic health. Equality and autonomy for patients is likewise important, as long as it does not suggest, as too often it does, an adversary relationship between holistic and orthodox medicine. Holistic health practices, like those of so many other aspects of alternative medicine, should not be thought of so much as alternative but as complementary, particularly as they emphasize the psychic and social aspects of medical care.

The notion that any kind of therapy, from homeopathy, chelation

74. James, W., *The varieties of religious experience.* New York: Modern Library, 1902, p. 94.

therapy, acupuncture, nutritional therapy, to clinical ecology and stress reduction can all deal equally with disease is one that no rational physician can accept. We are back with voodoo, folk medicine, and charlatanism. Touching and massage, and some of the other techniques, are all very good and clearly ways for the patient to feel (literally) that somebody out there cares. I rather suspect that they represent simply another form of psychotherapy, a form of placebo. But the large number of people coming to doctor's offices for whom high or low technology medicine has little to offer must account for the great interest in alternative medicine. In Britain, for example, more than 80 percent of physicians responding to a questionnaire wanted to explore at least one form of such an approach.

James's comments on "mind-cure" are pertinent one hundred years later:

> To the importance of mind-cure the medical and clerical professions in the United States are beginning, though with much recalcitrancy and protesting, to open their eyes. . . . The important point is that so large a number should exist who *can* be so influenced [by the mind-cure movement].[75]

In many ways looking at the placebo brings the question out in the open, forces the practitioner to recognize that it is *not* the ritual, nor the pill which has the power, but the practitioner—and the time he spends with the patient, the energy he directs at helping. The placebo has no power of its own; it is inert and inactive, but it is the person giving it who gives the help, the miracle of one person helping another.

The major problem lies in the claims that holistic medicine makes without observations. We need to return to the definitions of charlatanism. A charlatan pretends to possess secrets in the healing art. Certainly that is not true of most holistic medical practitioners, but a scientist tries to develop an organizing view and hypotheses which will explain his facts and observations which will test his hypotheses. For the charlatan there is no testing of experience or changing of hypotheses because of observations. That is, I think, where the holistic practitioners go astray.

Holistic physicians, no more than any others, too often do not discriminate clearly enough between disease and illness, as must be done to evaluate healing methods. The triumphs of treating illness presumably are the triumphs of changing the disorders of perception, and their techniques are the same placebo techniques with faith and other kinds of approaches that I have been examining here. Holistic practitioners have no recognized set of problems and no shared standards

75. Ibid.

for solutions, as Glymore and Stalker suggested in their indictment in the *New England Journal of Medicine* some years ago.[76]

In summary then, many of the goals of the holistic medical practitioners are congenial, but their claims for specific merit need not be taken seriously. We should judge the movement by the same scientific criteria we have used for the placebo. Scientists take data, see if they can reproduce and categorize it, and then, after they have asked whether it happens more than once, ask *why* it happens. Holistic practitioners have not done that and until they do, we need not believe that holistic medicine forms anything other than a more enthusiastic form of psychotherapy that is important and effective, but one for which no special claims can be made.

The question is whether the holistic approach, or any other form of what has become known as alternative medicine, has any special insights that would not be possessed by any prudent experienced practitioner. I cannot find such insights. To some extent its strengths come from its novelty in a scientific age, from the allure of the romantic. Novelty has always been effective in cure, whether by alternative or orthodox measures. The term *alternative* suggests an approach different from that of orthodox medicine. The emphasis is different so that the term *complementary* is more apt. There is no either-or. A balance is desirable. Alternative holistic practitioners treat the whole patient, emphasize the personal factors "in a direct and continuous dialogue between doctor and patient."[77] In a rational medical payment scheme intended to deemphasize the technological aspects of medical practice, physicians would be paid as much (or more) for the time spent *with* the patient as for the things done *to* the patient. That is the big task of alternative medicine, to benefit the illness, not the disease.

As so often in these matters, William James says much that is still applicable to our times:

> The obvious outcome of our total experience is that the world can be handled according to many systems of ideas, and is so handled by different men. . . . Science gives to all of us telegraphy, electric lighting, and diagnosis, and succeeds in preventing and curing a certain amount of disease. Religion in the shape of mind-cure gives to some of us serenity, moral poise, and happiness, and prevents certain forms of disease as well as science does, or even better in a certain class of persons.[78]

76. Glymour, C., and Stalker, D., Engineers, cranks, physicians, magicians, *NEJM* 308:960–64, 1983.

77. Lister, S., Current controversy on alternative medicine, *NEJM* 309:1524–27, 1983.

78. James, *The varieties of religious experience*, p. 120.

David Owen, a physician and British politician, suggests that holistic medicine can help to strike a better balance in medical care:

The holistic approach is not a new fangled, trendy manifestation of quirky and way-out opinions. It is the reassertion of the traditional medical values where a sensitivity to the individuality of the person is a precious part of the practice of the healing profession. The practice of medicine involves the whole person.[79]

The important question remains whether acupuncture, holistic medicine, or even psychotherapy achieve their ends by means of the specific technique credited or because of the amount of time spent with the patient. A little less than 60 percent of people felt "much better" after attending an alternative medical clinic for such nonspecific complaints as back or abdominal pain, feeling "run-down," or headaches, many of which had not been relieved by visits to conventional practitioners. That phenomenon must be telling us something.

Ironically the claims of alternative medicine are best attested to by William James himself. James had William Osler, then professor of medicine at Oxford, as friend and physician, but when James was sick, in 1910, eight years after the Gifford Lectures which formed the basis for his book on *The Varieties of Religious Experience*, James went off to an unknown physician in Paris whom he characterized as a "quack." He didn't even ask Osler's advice. He simply went.

On April 3, 1908, William James wrote in part to Osler, "I find myself in a state of as bad nervous fatigue as I have ever been in my life, and that says a good deal. Today, e.g., awake since 2.30 and had to stop work on my 5th lecture (out of 8) after two hours because of flushed head."[80] Later, on May 5, 1910, when his writer brother, Henry James, seventy-two was sick enough to be referred to as "the invalid," whose case was "more and more plainly one of melancolia," James told Osler that he was going off to Paris to see a Doctor Montier. In the same letter that he thanked Osler for advice he informed him of his decision: "I ought to tell you that your advice in my daughter's case . . . was fully corroborated by events." Nevertheless, he added:

My anginoid pain has increased during the past year, tho' nitroglycerin stops it like magic. I go to Paris to consult one Dr. Montier, whose high frequency currents have performed a *wunder kur* on a neighbor of mine. . . . I know of two cases of similar relief by him, tho' I am unacquainted with the details. It sounds impossible, and I

79. Owen, D., Medicine, morality, and the market. *Lancet* 2:30–31, 1984.
80. Edelstein, L., Appendix (Letters from William James to William Osler), *Bull. Hist. Med.* 20:292–93, 1946.

hear that M. is regarded as a quack by medical opinion. Nevertheless, I don't wish to leave that stone unturned, since my own trouble (in which I gladly acknowledge an element of nervous hyperaesthesia) seems progressive. I will let you know the results!

That a man whose opinion we still quote today should choose for himself a charlatan suggests the continuing need for romanticism in medicine.

11

Physicians' Resistance to the Placebo

Physicians in the past used placebos quite frequently, but an informal survey suggests that is certainly not the case today. Indeed, physicians now generally deny giving placebos, as if to do so would be putting something over on the patient. Deliberately using a placebo sometimes makes a physician feel guilty! Few pure placebos are handed out today. Instead physicians give impure placebos, to keep from admitting even to ourselves what we are doing.

Guilt at using placebos stems from: (1) medical school education based on the model of physics as *the* exact science, which most scholars have tried to emulate, and which in medicine goes by the term "the biomedical model." The now much-maligned Cartesian dualism of mind and body makes the body a machine and the brain a computer; (2) fear of being a charlatan, or at least being thought to be one. Maybe even more fear of having to face doubts about the scientific model, if the placebo is effective, of confronting the fact that the scientific model does not explain everything, also plays a role.

TRAINING OF PHYSICIANS

The Ancient Heritage

I have suggested that the physician looking at the placebo begins to bridge the chasm between the scientific, naturalistic, and rationalistic basis of all that has been achieved and the personalistic, priestly, irrational, romantic and even mystical heritage which he has attempted to deny. It is the conflict between the Enlightenment and the Romantics, the Counter-Enlightenment. Whether we look at folk

186

medicine anew or trace medical practice from the antipodes of Hippocrates and Aesculapius makes little difference.

From its beginnings medical practice has alternated between the two poles of reason and intuition, most recently in our Western society given the names of the Enlightenment and the Counter-Enlightenment.[1] No doubt I have wrenched some observations to fit prejudices, but the lens of the placebo has focused on these stresses.

So thorough has been our nurturing in the world of science that most doctors view medical history as one mighty climb away from intuition and Romanticism toward reason and science. They are quite unaware of countervailing forces because of their indoctrination. Partly that comes about because of the separation of medical life from intellectual life in the wider world and in the universities. Teachers in the medical school want to be seen as scientists, but not too many of them are anxious to be considered poets. It was not always that way. Until the twentieth century, whatever influenced intellectual history generally also played a large role in medical thought. From my vantage point it looks as if physicians were more active in intellectual life in the past than they are today. Maybe the change has come about because in the past physicians were among the educated few, whereas today far more people have gone to college.

In some ways medical practice and science at the end of the twentieth century, to use Toynbee's old term , look like a "fossil civilization," unchanged in viewpoint since the scientific revolution began.[2] Orthodox medicine has no room for Romanticism or intuition and enshrines only the ideas of the Enlightenment. Holistic storms can rage without, but the spaceship of molecular medicine soars on towards its goal. Psychoanalysis and psychiatry examine the intuitive emotional background of man, but many current psychiatrists are so anxious to prove themselves logical scientists (and if they are university professors to get funding) that they replace the mind with the brain. Neurobiology holds sway even in some psychiatric departments. Freud, to a great extent, was the romantic of our time even if he saw himself as a scientist, and the holistic movement, like the alternative medicine movement generally, represent the romantic reaction to the sway of reason.

The Enlightenment which enshrines Newton in physics brought on the inevitable counterreaction in the world outside medicine, but in medical practice Enlightenment ideals have never changed or yielded. The "medico-materialists" and reductionists have no room for complementary views. That is why man is seen by doctors as only

1. Berlin, I., *Against the current*. New York: Penguin, 1980.
2. Toynbee, A. J., *A study of history*. London: Oxford University Press, 1948.

his body. Only the body and its reactions and organs can be measured and photographed, "imaged" really.

This recurrent cycle of reactions goes unemphasized by all but a few medical historians. The history of medicine has often been written without enough attention to outside influences, particularly when it is written by physicians. Even in current medical journals ideas are often introduced as new without being put into context with the medical past. As I have remarked several times, sometimes in thinking about the placebo I have worried that I am simply writing about what is obvious and well known, but rereading a number of papers has convinced me that many commentators and critics offer their conclusions in too great isolation from what has been written earlier. Houston does not refer to William James, Engel ignores Houston, and so on. Many of us see ourselves as rebel angels with no relationship to Lucifer.

With the foregoing in mind, I will review a few highlights that are pertinent to looking at the placebo.

Greek medicine. The basis of Hippocratic medicine, so Castiglione tells us approvingly, was: (1) a wide knowledge of natural sciences; (2) profound experience in practical medicine; (3) clear and logical reasoning about cause and effect; and (4) ethical concepts. He sets this off against priestly or Aesculapian medicine which relied on (1) dreams, oracles, and miracles, and (2) the unreasonable caprices of the gods, and which therefore lacked a consistent underpinning of cause and effect.[3]

Castiglione suggests that Greek medicine "was not predominantly magic or priestly" (p. 120), even though it began as empirical craft which later became mystical and priestly. The cult of Aesculapius, whose serpent symbol has remained paradoxically enough the symbol of modern medicine, was introduced about 429 B.C. Temples to Aesculapius were built near the sea for their refreshing breezes and were adorned with works of art, much like many modern Western hospitals. Baths, abstinence, and ceremonies, so Castiglione tells us, interpretation of dreams and even hypnotic states, all formed part of the cure. Priestly medicine, according to all accounts, must have worked, but it was practiced exclusively by priests and "the cures were regarded as miraculous." We can believe that the whole setting of the healing scene must have been important: the magnificent situation of the temples, together with the "dietary measures, baths, and massage," enlarged the effect of the faith which the patients brought with

3. Castiglione, A., *A history of medicine.* New York: Knopf, 1947, pp. 148–78.

them. Castiglione regards the Aesculapian school with disdain, however effective it might have been for what I have called illness.

Edelstein, on the other hand, is not as quick to denigrate the religious and the magic in ancient Greek medicine.[4] Although he sees the Greek physicians as being rational and empirical, he finds them all influenced by religious ideas. Greek physicians as a whole, particularly the dogmatists, were hostile to magic, which they rejected as useless and wrong. But as he points out, "when the art of the physician fails, everybody resorts to incantation and prayers" (p. 245).

From their earliest Greek predecessors, physicians have, with various lapses, trained themselves to analyze logically from observed data and have based their treatments and their advances on such reproducible phenomena. Diagnosis, after all, depends upon being able to predict from what you hear and what you will see, and prognosis depends upon knowing that what has happened in the past will happen again. If there are no logical consequences, there can be no rational predictions. The Greek physicians were first of all empiricists and, like their modern heirs, distrusted revealed dogma. They also distrusted the patients, regarding what they had to say as mere opinion. Virgil, Entralgo tells us, for such reasons called medicine the "silent art."

For the physician, the *Iliad* offers a striking contrast between illnesses brought on by the whimsicality of the gods, which could only be changed by priests who sacrificed suitable hecatombs of animals, and the wounds of battle, which could be treated by laymen but which were better treated by physicians.[5] But if Apollo can bring on a plague capriciously, and if only sacrifices and other forms of propitiation can rid us of the plague, there is no need for the logical approach of the physician. A priest is needed for such matters. To a great extent physicians in the *Iliad* work largely as trauma surgeons, dressing wounds, staunching blood, and stopping pain.

The trivium and quadrivium. We learn from White that in the Middle Ages the seven liberal arts were divided into the trivium (grammar, rhetoric, and logic), which had to do with verbal methods of analysis, and the quadrivium (arithmetic, geometry, astronomy, and music), which dealt with measurement and calculation. Later, faith waned as the mathematic and physical sciences rose in estimate, and the trivium yielded in importance to the quadrivium. Galileo, Newton, and others

4. Edelstein, L., The professional ethics of the Greek physician, *Bull. Hist. Med.* 30:391–419, 1956.

5. Homer, *The Iliad*, Robert Fitzgerald, New York: Anchor, 1975.

seemed to prove the all-encompassing importance of the quadrivium. Yet White exhorts us

> What must be denied is that mathematics, measurement, and quantification provide much insight into the deepest personal problems and experiences of our race: courage and cowardice, affection and hatred, generosity and greed, charm and repulsion, courtesy and boorishness, awe and mockery. . . . About such matters we can only talk to each other, at length, carefully, trivially. We must talk patiently, weighing contradictions, balancing paradoxes, and not expecting to arrive at 'laws' but rather at rough consensus that draws on long experience and takes a long view of the road ahead. Quadrivial ways are useful, but those who employ them habitually because they produce good harvest from their special fields must recognize more vividly the severe limitations of their favorite method.[6]

The Enlightenment

To some extent the emphasis on quantification is a modern phenomenon. The Enlightenment was responsible for the current faith that techniques applied in astronomy and physics can give rational answers to all problems.

The Enlightenment was that remarkable period of the eighteenth century in which faith in science and particularly confidence in progress to ultimate perfectability led to the expectation that the scientific method, which had achieved such triumphs in the world of physics, could do the same for all fields of human endeavor—social, literary, and spiritual among them. The principles of the Enlightenment cannot be encapsulated in a brief paragraph. Isaiah Berlin describes the central principles of the Enlightenment as "universality, objectivity, rationality, and the capacity to provide permanent solutions to all genuine problems of life or thought, and (not less important) accessibility or rational methods to any thinker armed with adequate powers of observation and logical thinking."

Berlin describes how the Enlightenment adopted mathematics as the "science of sciences." He traces that back to Plato, but the contrast between reason which measures and intuition which grasps in a flash has been traced back farther than the Greeks. Shryock notes that drugs were widely measured in ancient Egypt and that in Alexandria in the third century B.C. attempts to measure physiological behavior were common.

6. White, L., Technical assessment from the stance of a medical historian, *Amer. Hist. Rev.* 79:1–13, 1974.

THE COUNTER-ENLIGHTENMENT

The Counter-Enlightenment came along as a reaction to the rational logical approach of the physicists and it culminated in the Romantic movement of the nineteenth century. The Counter-Enlightenment was the reaction to what Berlin has called the "autonomy of reason and the methods of natural sciences based on observation as the sole reliable method of knowledge and the consequent rejection of the authority of revelation, sacred writings and their accepted interpreters, tradition, prescription, and every form of non-rational and transcendent source of knowledge."[7]

Was there a unified organized intellectual opposition which deserved to be called a counter-revolution or *the* Counter-Enlightenment? Historians of intellectual thought suggest that the Counter-Enlightenment probably never comprised a unified group, but a number of people thought alike and influenced each other.[8] Although he was not widely read in his time, scholars have traced the modern beginnings of the Counter-Enlightenment to Vico of Naples in the early eighteenth century. He saw cycles in cutural development, not the ever-advancing spiral we all think of today. For Vico each culture was unique, its questions and answers unique and not to be compared to those of another culture in a different setting. Vico sounds like the best candidate for the patron saint of medical anthropology. His notion that symbols mean different things at different times to different men could prove relevant to thinking about the placebo. Hamann of Konisberg had a theological background with a faith in God which made him ultimately believe that religious experience and personal inner life were more important than the truth of the senses. Herder suggested that societies had to be understood in terms of their own structure and cultural heritage.

The Romantic movement, for our purposes at least, was equivalent to the Counter-Enlightenment and was the culmination of the reaction to the rule of rationality, but Romanticism hardly touched medical practice. To explore the differences between Rationalism and Romanticism in medicine, we can look at the rejection of the Enlightenment principle of universality, objectivity, and rationality as characteristic of "alternative medicine." Baumer gives us a useful definition of Romanticism: "Romanticism might better be said to have centered

7. Berlin, I., The Counter-Enlightenment, in *Dictionary of Historical Ideas*, vol. 2., New York: Scribner, 1973, pp. 100–12.

8. Ibid.; Wellek, R., Romanticism in literature, in *Dictionary of the History of Ideas*, vol. 2, New York: Scribner, 1973, pp. 187–98; Baumer, F. L., Romanticism, in ibid., pp. 198-204.

in several quite marked predispositions: an emphasis on particularity or individuality, and a sense of the infinite and the irrational component in human life."[9] While scholars like Lovejoy have pointed out that "the word 'romantic' has come to mean so many things that by itself it means nothing,"[10] physicians need not unduly concern themselves with the problems of historians in categorizing different movements and in putting boundaries to them. We physicians simply need to see that the struggles, if the unequal balance between medical reductionists and counterreductionists today can even be called a struggle, has its origin in the intellectual currents of the rest of society.

Man lives in two worlds: he has a body and he has a mind. The mind is more than the brain, and it would be as foolhardy to emphasize the tenets of alternative medicine in treating only the mind as it would be to emphasize the tenets of rational science and emphasize only the body. There is a place for both neurobiology and psychiatry. For us the Counter-Enlightenment and Romanticism suggest that we physicians need to recognize men as men and not only as collections of organs, men as willing their destinies, each unique with strivings and even higher purposes with deep feelings and intuitions.

I review this problem to emphasize that the struggles of the moment need to be seen in the light of the traditions from which they spring even if the people writing about them seem to have little concept of their origins.

MEDICAL EDUCATION IN THE UNITED STATES

To a large extent we can trace the resistance to the placebo to the modern training of physicians, something which was standardized for the United States by the Flexner report of 1910, his enduring contribution to medical education.[11]

Flexner surveyed 150 medical schools at a time when there had been an enormous overproduction of "uneducated and ill-trained medical practitioners"; a tide of "unprepared youth is drawn out of industrial occupations into the study of medicine" for the sake of profit. Flexner gave very specific comments about each medical school in the United States. To read his report is to learn how bad medical education was. Nevertheless, one has to read Flexner in his time.

I am not suggesting that the Flexner report alone was responsible

9. Baumer, Romanticism.
10. Lovejoy, A. O., quoted in Baumer, Romanticism.
11. Flexner, A., *Medical education in the United States and Canada*, New York: Carnegie Foundation, 1910.

for reductionism in medical education and practice in the United States. Hired to provide a disinterested, impartial, (and possibly predictable) view of medical education, to a large extent Flexner simply crystallized reports and ideas which were already current. Forces promoting science were as powerful outside the United States as within, and it would be too chauvinistic to suggest that the Flexner report influenced medical practice throughout the world. I simply suggest that for American medical education the Flexner report effectively silenced consideration of what could *not* be reduced to "facts" and measure.

As King has pointed out, emphasizing science in medical school involves two quite different and "potentially contradictory philosophies."[12] The training of medical practitioners and the expansion of medical knowledge are not necessarily well done by the same institution or, at least, by the same people. Training of practitioners was classically the function of medical education, expansion of knowledge the province of the university.

It may not be an overstatement to find that Flexner's disdain of theory or preconceptions and his overestimation of "facts" and the scientific methods still largely dominate medical thinking today. A man of the Enlightenment, he had no tolerance for what was not "scientific." So near as I can tell, current notions of scientific discovery, which place a great emphasis on theory dominating the "facts" that are discovered have had little influence in the way medical educators and therefore physicians look at matters. Physicists may think that the uncertainty principle dominates quantum mechanics, and may suggest that the same unpredictability shapes the millions of neural connections in the brain, but that uncomfortable randomness has not weakened the clinician's ideal of the "hard-wired" brain.

For Flexner, whose thinking has so dominated American medical education ever since, there were three stages in the evolution of medical teaching. His objectives and time spans are different, and as a scientist his notions are very different from those of Jewson, but we can glimpse the same three stages: (1) the patient in a bed, (2) the case in a hospital, and (3) the assemblage of organs and systems in a body.

The first stage for Flexner was the era of dogma, from Hippocrates through Galen down to the sixteenth century. Hippocrates had begun with empirical observation and his own experience, but succeeding generations of practitioners who followed his teaching were dominated by scholasticism rather than by their own observations.

12. King, L. S., The Flexner Report of 1910, *JAMA* 251:1079–86, 1984.

The second era was that of the empiric in the sixteenth century, which

at its best it leaned upon experience, but its means of analyzing, classifying, and intepreting phenomena were painfully limited. Medical art was still under the sway of preconceived and preternatural principles of explanation; and rigorous therapeutic measures were not uncommonly deduced from purely metaphysical assumptions.

The third era is the scientific one:

Medicine is part and parcel of modern science. The human body belongs to the animal world. It is put together of tissues and organs, and their structure, origin, and development not essentially unlike what the biologist is otherwise familiar with. . . . We may then fairly describe modern medicine as characterized by a severely critical handling of experience. It is at once more skeptical and more sure than mere empiricism. For though it takes nothing on faith, the fact which it accepts does not fear the hottest fire. (pp. 52–53)

Knowledge "procured" is what is accepted, not knowledge "received":

The sectarian, on the other hand, begins with his mind made up. He possesses in advance a general formula, which the particular instance is going to illustrate, verify, reaffirm, even though he may not know just how. One may be sure that facts so read will make good what is expected of them; that only that will be seen which will sustain its expected functions; that every aspect noted will be dutifully loyal to the revelation in whose favor the observer is predisposed: the human mind is so constituted.

In contrast, the scientist or physician finds knowledge in the future: "It is precisely the function of scientific method . . . to get rid of such hinderances to clear thought and effective action. For it, comprehensive summaries are situated in the future, not in the past; we shall attain them, if at all, at the end of great travail; they are not lightly to be assumed prior to the beginning" (pp. 156–57).

Facts were more important than theories, and in his attempt to get rid of the medical sects he wrote, "It needs theories only as convenient summaries in which a number of ascertained facts may be used tentatively to define a course of action."

Flexner saw the acquisition of knowledge as getting one fact after another, in order to avoid any preconceived notions. Yet when he talks of the difference between empiric medicine and scientific medicine, it is hard to discern all the differences. As he saw it the difference between the empiric and the scientific was that theory followed facts in the scientific mode, but preceded them in the empirical mode. Not many philosophers of science would agree with him today, but the notion that a theory is built on the painstaking acquisition of "facts" or "observations" is still congenial to his medical heirs today who believe even today that "facts accumulate faster than theories can accommodate them."[13]

Curiously enough in contrast to current enthusiasm for family practice, Flexner did not want to train two kinds of physicians, those who would become scientists to do research and those who would become family doctors. He believed that bedside practice required a working hypothesis fully as much as laboratory investigation.

I looked in vain in Flexner's report for an understanding of the patient himself. Chapter 2 is as close as we get:

> The practitioner deals with facts of two categories. Chemistry, physics, biology enable him to apprehend one set; he needs a different apperceptive and appreciative apparatus to deal with the other, more subtle elements. Specific preparation is in this direction much more difficult; one must rely for the requisite insight and sympathy on a varied and enlarging cultural experience.
>
>   It goes without saying that this type of doctor is first of all an educated man. (p. 26)

We should not criticize Flexner for not seeing further. He did not need to worry about the physician's being a cultured or an educated man. His task was to clean the stables. Within ten years of his report many "nonscientific" medical schools had closed and the view of the physician as scientist collecting facts had begun its reign, to this day.

The placebo has provided our lens to look at the tensions between reason and intuition. We have seen that physicians live in two worlds: the world of science which provides them with their knowledge of disease, with very real advances against disease, and with their current ideals. But they also live in the world of people, with instincts, pain, suffering, hope, and joy. The first is the universe of physics, the other is the realm of the poet.

Margulis states it differently, as befits a philosopher: "Medicine is primarily an art and, dependently, a science. It is primarily an institutionalized service concerned with the care and cure of the ill and the control of disease. . . . Medicine is a doubly normative discipline."[14]

13. Medawar, P. S., Two conceptions of science, in *The art of the soluble*, London: Methuen, 1967, p. 115.

14. Margulis, J., The concept of disease, *J. Med. Phil.* 1:238–55, 1976.

That world of the physicist, however, has provided the most attractions for physicians who look on the humanities as providing refreshment but little education. They have embraced the scientific fallacy.

Scientific Fallacy

In large part modern resistance to the use of the placebo comes from the "scientific fallacy" that most physicians have accepted. What characterizes the current era of medical thinking is the faith that all matters can be solved by quantitation. The *reductionists* is one pejorative term often used for the same people William James called "medico-materialists."[15] In passing, it is worthwhile noting, however, that medical practice is not alone in embracing this scientific fallacy. Anthropologists, sociologists, psychologists, and members of most other learned professions seem to have accepted the idea that the techniques of the hard sciences will give them answers that are permanent and comparable. More important, they have the idea that giving a number to something makes their answers scientific. Some young scholars may disagree with their elders in this regard, but to get promoted and to flourish, they have to measure something.

Wittgenstein comments:

> Our craving for generality has another main source: Our preoccupation with the method of science. I mean the method of reducing the explanation of natural phenomena to the smallest possible number of primitive natural laws; and, in mathematics, of unifying the treatment of different topics by using a generalization. Philosophers constantly see the method of science before their eyes, and are irresistably tempted to ask and answer questions in the way science does. This tendency is the real source of metaphysics, and leads the philosopher into complete darkness.[16]

Along with many other learned professionals, physicians have come to believe that (1) measurement and quantification are essential to knowledge; and that (2) facts and observations are entirely objective. In looking to molecular biology for the answers to pain and suffering, they mistake the part for the whole. In a flight from their Aesculapian heritage (even though it may go unrecognized), to avoid being thought charlatans, they avoid anything that smacks of intuition. The clinician used to attend to the needs of his patients while the pathologist or biochemist looked at the function of organs and their biochemical abnormalities. Now that training has distorted the clincian's values, he too prefers to look at the smaller units.

15. James, W., *Varieties of religious experience,* New York, Modern Library, 1902, p. 14.
16. Wittgenstein, L., *The blue and brown books,* New York: Harper and Row, 1965, p. 18.

It is easy to see why. Physicians treat persons in whom personal, social, and psychological components influence manifestations of disease. Looking around, they do not find great advances in the understanding of "man" or of "society." When they study disease processes in which quantification has been responsible for major advances, they conclude that scientific methods offer the only triumphs. Physicians nowadays know so much more about lupus than about lust, that they cannot be blamed for believing that quantification should yield answers even to desire.

Over the past one hundred years advances in medical practice have come about because of the scientific method devoted to the study of disease and the processes which engender it. Shryock has emphasized how scientific and therefore medical management has advanced much faster in areas where quantification has been reliable than in areas where quantification has not been possible. The temptation, therefore, is to measure what you can, and let the rest go. The security of objective data is hard to abandon. The gaze of the physician-scientist has, therefore, focused on smaller and smaller bits; from person and symptom, to organ and disease, to cell and pathophysiology, and finally to subcellular particles and genetic engineering. The clinician no longer wonders why physics rather than poetry should hold his attention. Painstaking measurement, testing of hypotheses by exciting new technology, have brought such enormous clinical rewards. The scientific method has put the quietus for physicians on anything that smacks of intuition, mysticism, or irrationality. Repression, as Alexander put it, is the defense:

The aversion to the introduction of psychologic factors in medicine is due to the fact that it reminds the physicians of those not very remote days in which medicine was sorcery, and therapy consisted of expelling the evil demons from the body. Medicine, this newcomer among the exact sciences, has the typical mentality of all newcomers. It tries to make one forget its dark, magical past and therefore it has to watch out carefully that nothing suspicious should remain in it which could betray these undesirable remnants of its prescientific period. Physics, this aristocrat of the natural sciences, can better afford to overthrow its basic principles and undergo a profound reorientation, whereas medicine feels it necessary to emphasize its exact nature in keeping out of its field everything that seems to endanger its scientific appearance. Indeed, among the exact sciences medicine became more pope-like than the Pope himself.[17]

17. Alexander, F., Functional disturbances of psychogenic nature, *JAMA* 100: 409–73, 1933.

Science, of course, can be simply the symbol or ritual by which physicians keep uncertainty at a distance. The laboratory reports levels in the blood to two or three decimal points to give an aura of accuracy to medical practice. Working in a laboratory during training on experiments which can be tightly controlled trains the young physician to believe that precise measurements bring certainty. The men and women who leave for clinical practice keep that training for precision in their hearts and regret that they have abandoned the search for truth.

Having taken for their domain all illness and disease as historical developments have put licensing of medical care in the hands of the physicians, modern physicians don't quite know what to do with illness. When there was a more general and eclectic approach in the mid-nineteenth century, many complaints were handled outside the medical offices and responded quite well, as the Emmanuel Movement suggested. The problem is that once having taken over all human complaints as their field of action, doctors trained to deal with diseases from the scientific approach tend to look at illness with the same tools and approaches.

Measurement and Quantification

Medical students and practicing physicians sometimes are in despair at all the facts and numbers they are supposed to keep in their heads. Without some grasp of historical developments they may assume that the esteem in which quantification is currently held is a new phenomenon. That may lead them to imagine the good old days were different. Many medical students have said to me something like, "I went to medical school to learn to take care of patients. I think I have something to offer, that as a physician I can be more of a person, more of a care-taker than many doctors that I have seen. Yet, as near as I can tell, medicine and medical practice focus on numbers and quantification."

Two kinds of knowledge. In ancient Greece, Shryock tells us, knowledge was of two kinds, measuring and nonmeasuring.[18] There was a specific kind of knowledge in cybernetics and statistics, but the physician who was (at that time at least) necessarily less precise stood for the other kind of knowledge, using his human qualities without numbers. (We should not forget that the physician was the model of government for Aristotle and other philosophers.) Quantification fell into decline, as far as medical practice was concerned, however, Shryock

18. Shryock, R. H., The history of quantification in medical science, *Isis*, 52: 215–37, 1961.

suggests, partly because the phenomena which could be measured were not yet recognized and partly, and more important, because the intellectual climate of the time favored the nonmeasuring approach. Taxonomy—classification and description—was more important than measurement.

You only know what you can count. Later, when Newton became the model of the intellectual, the objectivist tradition began to hold sway. Objective knowledge and objective truth were its goal. There were three basic assumptions according to Berlin: (1) every genuine question has one true answer and one only; (2) a rational, logical method will lead to correct solutions in all problems; and (3) there are true universal, eternal and immutable laws. Especially in the seventeenth and eighteenth centuries men built systems based on rational insight and mathematical reasoning, put their faith in controlled observation and experiment in the belief that there was only one true method. That was, after all, he emphasizes, "the hour of the greatest triumph of the natural sciences." Goethe warned, however, that measurement could be employed in strictly physical sciences, but that biological, psychological, and social phenomena eluded quantitation and abstraction. But the ways of the natural scientist triumphed. More important, the philosophers agreed that logic and rationality could give the right answers.

What followed, through logical positivism and the Vienna Circle to the present day, has played "a decisive role in the social, legal and technological organization of our world." Certainly there is no place where this is better exemplified than late twentieth-century medical practice. The scientific model strongly implies that " only that which was quantifiable, or at any rate measurable . . . was real." As William James put it, "The aim of 'science' is to attain conceptions so adequate and exact that we shall never need to change them."[19]

I need not trace how this view has come to dominate medicine so much that physicians have forgotten their place in the world of persons and have an eye only for the world of diseases. Physicians should think about how much their concepts have been restricted by science. To a large extent scientists stand at the borders of the unknown looking ahead; technicians look backward to measure what is predictable, and so look backward. Technology is steady, measuring what is predictably already known, moving solidly ahead. Medical research to a large extent passes only the technology test. Knowledge advances the most when scientists find phenomena which challenge current theories and which do not seem to fit them. Kuhn has one view of the process: the scientist says, "Well, I don't know why this should happen.

19. James, *Varieties of religious experience.*

According to our theories, it doesn't make sense, but here it is! Therefore, let's look into the matter, revise our theories and try to figure
out why." For Popper or Kuhn science advances by testing concepts.
Lewin tells us that for Cassirer

> The basic character of science. . . . [is]. . . . the eternal attempt to go
> beyond what is regarded scientifically accessible at any specific
> time. To proceed beyond the limitation of a given level of knowl-
> edge the researcher, as a rule, has to break down methodological
> taboos which condemn as "unscientific" or "illogical" the very
> methods or concepts which later on prove to be basic for the next
> major progress.[20]

Indeed, in the *New England Journal*, in 1983 two engineers emphasized the model of physician as engineer. "People need to be understood as causal systems very much as do bridges and boats and air
planes and bacteria. Without understanding people as objects in this
way, there can be no such thing as medical science."[21]

It is more than just landing a man on the moon or putting a mechanical heart in an old dentist or a baboon's in a baby. The rational
principles of the Enlightenment, the belief that goes back to Plato,
suggests that "truth" is discoverable by logic and that there are underlying structures and general principles which enough study will let us
discern, for all time. This has been the main controlling theme of
Western thought for at least several hundred years. Reason, logic,
and science are the main ingredients of physician's education. The
notion that there might be a medicine specifically Chinese or Greek
or, in terms of ten or fifteen years ago, a black medicine, seems farfetched to him. The enzymes, genes, and cells function in the human
body all in about the same way. The idea that ethnic, cultural, or emotional differences play a role in illness or in the response to it seems to
many physicians only a temporary, even repugnant, aberration which
the triumph of science will eliminate.

A good example is how physicians study the patient whose ulcer is
refractory to treatment with the latest agents. They increase the dos-
ages of the H2 blockers, change the forms of medical therapy, talk of
operations, and run statistical trials of how operations affect such patients. Yet neither acid levels nor demographic characteristics seem to
account for the fact that 10 to 15 percent of patients do not respond
to therapy, endoscopically at least. Physicians ignore the fact that the
ulcers may give no clinical symptoms when they recur and, more as-

20. Lewin, K., *Field theory in social science*, New York: Harper, 1964.
21. Glymour, C., and Stalker, D., Engineers, cranks, physicians, magicians, *NEJM*
308:960–64, 1983.

tonishingly, most physicians ignore psychological features which may contribute to the recurrence of such an ulcer. The ulcer is the target, along with the bad habits of the patient such as smoking, but his thoughts and stresses are virtually ignored.

What is a charlatan? I have said that no physician wants to be thought a fraud or charlatan, what used to be called a quack. According to the *OED*, a charlatan is "an empiric who pretends to possess secrets esp. in the healing art; an empiric or imposter in medicine, a quack." A major difference between a charlatan and a medical scientist in large part lies in the way in which they examine their experience, techniques, and results. The charlatan claims a hidden or magical power, mysteries arising from his person or his special knowledge, not to be understood by outsiders, whereas the scientist claims only what he has observed and measured. The scientist tries to develop an organizing view, hypotheses which will explain his facts, or observations which will test his hypotheses. For the charlatan or quack there is no testing of experience, certainly no changing of hypotheses because observations contradict them. Physicians have been trained as scientists.

Yet physicians cannot avoid looking at alternative approaches if only because laymen are so intrigued by them. Even though physicians have no wish to question the legitimacy or sufficiency of the scientific approach, still, they must look, at the nonrational forces in human nature and in human suffering, something which the revelations of psychiatry and psychoanalysis, of poetry and the humanities, have helped us to understand.

The two hurdles: Science and residency. The scientific fallacy has been responsible for the two major hurdles of medicine. The first is the hurdle of science, in college. To be eligible for medical school, the would-be physician must do very well in chemistry, physics, and other scientific disciplines. In his later professional life he may use that knowledge no more than any other educated person, but that hurdle must first be leaped. I sometimes think the reason has a religious base: it testifies to the fundamental loyalty to science that the physician must affirm. The second hurdle is the hospital-based residency. Nowadays this has become very technical, and as I have already described, such emphasis on high-technology, though crucial to the success of hospital care, bears little relationship to what the practitioner does in professional life later. Still, that hurdle must also be cleared. I doubt that the dilemmas of cost control and overreliance on technology in medicine will be resolved until physicians and educators ask themselves whether these two hurdles are as relevant as they once seemed.

ARE FACTS AND OBSERVATIONS
ALL THAT OBJECTIVE?

Physicians forget, because they have been so trained, how relativistic is even fact-finding. Outside the medical schools, increasing awareness of (1) the perceptual baggage that the scientist brings with him and (2) how culture and our preconceptions determine what we will see and what we will study makes "objectivity" seem less certain.

In almost all fields it seems that the preconceptions we bring along influence what we see, what we find, and what we do. It comes as no great surprise to find, for example, that lawyers have no very solid notion of "law" as something discoverable, but rather have the concept of the law as created, determined by culture and society. Philosophers will no doubt always try to arrive at a universal ethic, but pragmatists argue that culture determines what is, temporarily, ethical. Science is no different.

Wittengenstein emphasizes how much seeing is not really "seeing" as it is "seeing as." When I look at an ulcer crater, I don't say that I see a white spot with depth and a little redness around it, but rather I immediately see it as an ulcer crater because of other experiences that I have had and because of concepts with which I agree. The lack of objectivity of such an approach should be evident.

"Nature imitates art," said Oscar Wilde, in three words encapsulating a theory. Art historians have long pointed out how the artist's representation distorts reality for the viewer. Once someone has studied a painting, any later contrast with reality still leaves him accepting the artist's view as the best reality. We see what we are trained to see, and we understand best what proves our preconceptions. The savage before a word processor would see the keys as well as the student, but he could not put them into a context, would not really know what he saw. Seeing my wife and me hunched over a game called "Pente," my son, who had never seen the game before, could not at first interpret the meaning of the white and the red beads. Then, watching our moves, he recognized from his knowledge of Go what we were doing. Was that simply induction? Did his experience with Go help him select the observations to interpret? Theories precede data collection and influence what is collected rather than the other way around. There are so many facts and observations that we should be lost without some preconceptions. As Medawar puts it, "We cannot browse over the field of nature like cows at pasture."[22]

Einstein told Heisenberg, "On principle, it is quite wrong to try

22. Medawar, P. S., *Induction and intuition in scientific thought*, Philadelphia: American Philosophical Society, 1969, p. 29.

founding a theory on observable magnitudes alone. In reality the very opposite happens. It is the theory which decides what we can observe. You must appreciate that observation is a very complicated process. The phenomenon under observation produces certain events in our measuring apparatus."[23]

Induction and Deduction

To a large extent, I think, medical personnel accept the inductive method of science as the major one, though philosophers and others have emphasized that, as Medawar so nicely puts it, "Inductivism in scientific papers (is) simply the postures we choose to be seen in when the curtain goes up and the public sees us."

Induction is arguing from the "particular to the general," whereas *deduction* is arguing from the "general to the particular"; induction is the development of a theory from a set of facts. "Induction insists on the primacy of facts," but, as Medawar puts it, "Scientists select out facts to build their theories or probably more properly to buttress them." Physicians are trained in induction, or think they are. At least since Flexner in the United States, the primacy of facts and observations has gone unchallenged.

Importance of Intuition

Many scientists have talked of intuition, even some as scrupulously scientific as Medawar. An idea occurs unbidden, sudden and entire. Surely this could play a part in the healing as well as in the creative process? Why then should medicine be different? Medical practice has so recently emerged from the days of faith healing when physicians could do so little that we are afraid to be swept back. Yet a view of medical practice as much more than molecular biology, that man is more than a collection of chemicals, still appeals to many physicians. Is all thought really reducible to brain events? Medical practice should take into more account the social, psychological, and even spiritual dimensions of man. It is not that the scientific method misleads, but that it is misapplied.

Science as Religion

Feyerabend, a polemical writer known for his "anarchistic" theory of knowledge in his discussions of medicine, at least, makes a number of unwarranted and undocumented assumptions. Nevertheless he makes useful observations about the dogmatic character of science and the scientific method: no longer is it possible to question the sci-

---

23. Heisenberg, W., *Physics and beyond: Encounters and conversation*, New York: Harper, 1972, p. 63.

entific method because we are all indoctrinated in it. The citizen has the right to decide whether his child will be taught religion, but has no choice as to whether the child will be taught the scientific method, physics, and astronomy, for example. Feyerabend suggests that science should be looked at as part of our society, part of the way to understand nature, but he asserts that the idea that there is no knowledge outside science is nothing but a "fairy tale." Even metaphysical propositions may be important for medical practice: "A science that insists on possessing the only correct method and the only acceptable results is ideology."[24]

I will not recount Feyerabend's remarkable views of medicine. I agree with him that scientific chauvinism has no place in a profession which in its day to day actions deals with people much more than with diseases. As he puts it, "Voodoo has a firm though still not sufficiently understood material basis, and a study of its manifestations can be used to enrich, and perhaps even to revise, our knowledge of physiology." What he is saying, I think, is that all observations are still worth testing. That is what we have been looking at in relation to the placebo, and although Feyerabend might not accept that all observations should be tested by the scientific method, physicians can do little else. We may decide that some hypotheses deserve testing first and that some can be safely ignored. But we cannot ignore myths, dreams, and many other experiences even though we may differ from Feyerabend in how we evaluate them. In this regard, Jung makes the point that, "If, for instance, a general belief existed that the river Rhine had at one time flooded backwards from its mouth to its source, then this belief would in itself be a fact."[25]

Science need not become a religion and the only source of inspiration for physicians. We physicians need to approach our patients with fewer preconceptions. Molecular biology has remarkably advanced a specific segment of our understanding and treatment, but not all suffering has yielded to it. Because bacteria or viruses cause pneumonia, an invader does not also cause everything else. The triumphs of molecular biology over the past few years have been responsible for prolonging life and curing diseases. Yet that need not blind us to the observations that much of medical practice has little to do with science. Many physicians want to be regarded, by themselves and by others, as intellectuals, when in fact their skills arise in large part from other springs.

24. Feyerabend, P., *Against method: Outline of an anarchistic theory of knowledge*, London: Verso, 1978.

25. Jung, C., *Answer to Job*. New York: Meridian, 1964, p. 14.

ONE APPROACH

Medical education since Flexner has emphasized only the scientific measuring aspects of knowledge and has ignored such social sciences as anthropology or sociology which do not always bring statistical quantifications, or if they do, deal with aggregations of people that are too big for reductionists. The metaphor keeps changing, but it is always an active one: the physician *procures* information, *discovers* facts, *fights* disease, *finds* something new, always *deals* with something out there. Medical practice has followed the objectivist idea of the nineteenth-century rationalist. Psychiatry bloomed during the late nineteenth and early twentieth centuries, uncovering new dimensions to man's mental side. Now, however, even psychiatrists have become reductionists because the only way that they can regain respect from their colleague physicians is to become factual and biochemical.

One of the problems in medical ethics is that physicians have no very clear concept of what they mean by "man" or even by a "human being." In this we mirror the rest of society, but since physicians must study people and their diseases, it is too bad that we don't discuss such issues more. In our rounds and meetings we could have more fruitful discussions about *disease, illness, health, pain,* and the *patient*; we could argue whether we have made disease into an entity or whether the only thing that counts is how the person with the disease feels about it and reacts to it. We can let lawyers and judges and ethicists tell us when someone on a respirator is dead, but we ought to talk about these matters more among ourselves. Many ethical conflicts about treatment and diagnosis to a large extent, depend upon the fact that we do not very clearly examine "man" as the subject of our daily activities. We may try to define health and illness, but in our discussions of whom to keep alive, who to give our scarce resources to, and many more, we come down to the fact that until we agree on what a person is we will not arrive at any answers.

Take the issue of abortion. We do not agree on what to call the contents of the uterus. Proponents of abortion call those contents "the fetus" even just before term, but their foes refer to the "unborn child" almost from conception. These definitions are important, and although those having to do with abortion are fraught with religious concerns, physicians in general need to discuss their own working definitions of "man," "person," and many other ideas much more than we have. Until we do so, we can come to very few useful conclusions. I do not suggest that there are definitive answers that we will ever all agree on, but that the continuing discussion will help us sharpen our ideas.

The reader who is a physician may at once retort that such "soft" arguments are exactly what he wants to avoid, and such a physician would be following the usual lines of modern medical practice. Looking at what new has been learned about the mind, the physician feels quite justified in his approach. Freud aside, how little different is our understanding of human nature today than one hundred years ago? If a twenty-year period can move us from a state of helplessness in treating heart disease to the miracles of heart transplant and mechanical hearts, then surely such victories are but the forerunner of what science will someday teach us about character.

Medical Education: Tailors and Physicians

The training of physicians has followed an undeviating path since the Flexner report swept away alternate forms of therapy and codified the scientific approach to medicine. But the situation might be analogous to training someone to be a tailor by saying, "To become a tailor, you must first study polyester chemistry. Then it will be important to study the molecular structure of wool, to learn how sheep raised in different climates produce different kinds of wool. Later you will study how cotton grows, when it is best to pick it, and you will learn how its fibers are twisted to make yarn. For a year you will work in a factory making cloth and only then, after you have mastered all the fundamentals, you can go out and make clothes. When will you learn to make a suit? You will learn by doing!" Such a tailor might not sew a very fine seam, however grounded he might be in the basic science of tailoring.

Clinicians and medical educators will no doubt accept with only a little enthusiasm the analogy of a physician and a tailor, claiming that there is much more to medicine than technology. But then we will turn to them and say, "Where is your discussion of the patient as a person, of morals, of history that you say is so important?"

Hospital training for clinical practice. Is the analogy to medical education really so far off? After the medical student has graduated from medical school, he trains for three or four years in a hospital taking care of very sick patients. He becomes enormously skilled at activities which he will rarely or never do again or which will form a very small part of his tasks. A chief of cardiology remarked to me not too long ago how glad he was to spend a month as the "coronary care attending" because in that way he got the chance, once or twice a year, to "catch up" on what was new. Some years ago a resident in internal medicine told me how nervous she was about going back to that same coronary care unit because "now they unload the left ventricle, and I don't know how to do that!" The technology of medicine moves on so very fast that what is done one year is quickly outmoded the next. As a gastroenterologist I am not always sure that such frenzied activity denotes progress, and I fear that some of what passes for advance is simply fad, but still, routines (they are too kaleidoscopic to be called "customs") change almost yearly.

Physicians and hospitals have begun to welcome the idea that matters are so complicated that there must be specialists in emergency care or intensive care units, and in many other areas. Yet residents in medicine training for what will largely be office practice spend much of this time dealing with acute emergencies and the high technology that requires. They implicitly learn to look on patients as a collection of diseases to be acted upon. That was appropriate thirty or forty years ago, when practicing physicians were expected to care for sick patients in the neighborhood hospital. Now that hospital activities are so specialized, we need to ask whether such education prepares the physician for dealing with a patient in pain, someone with chronic disease, or for exploring the byways along which we are now traveling. In primitive cultures religion and medical practice may be one, but the wry observer in the West notes with Feyerabend that for most physicians science has become a religion from which we can deviate only at great cost.

The scientific, rational approach which depends upon controlled observation, and specifically upon the techniques of measuring, mathematics, and physics, has been the origin of much that has been worthwhile in medicine. Yet surely just as mental events are more than brain events, the informed imagination so cherished by the romantic movement of the Counter-Enlightenment, plays some role in human life and in human illness. The triumphs of the placebo may prove largely symbolic in origin, but that will be no less a victory. The physician lives, as I have emphasized, in two worlds: in the world of rational scientific logical achievement, drugs cure pneumonia; but in the other more instinctual, mythical world of sorrow and happiness, comforting and persuasive words, symbols, even only a reminder of the physician or of the healer, have power. Some attention to that world is surely not out of place in medical training because it plays so large a role in medical practice.

The medical student should study science, logic, mathematics to become expert in rational medicine, but reading history, fiction, and poetry will tell him something of the "trivial" other side. More important even, study of the humanities in medical school and in practice will not detract from his acquisition of the "data base" as much as it will let him look at charged issues with detachment and calm. Medical students and residents need reminders that man is more than his biology and that medical practice is more than biochemistry. The conflict between reason and logic on the one hand, and the unspoken and intuitive on the other, has always attended the healing arts.

It is a good sign that the American Board of Internal Medicine has begun to look at the humanistic qualities that physicians should have. They list them as integrity, respect, and compassion. Integrity is defined as the personal commitment to be honest and trustworthy in evaluating and demonstrating one's own skills and abilities. Respect is the personal commitment to honor others' choices and rights regarding themselves and their medical care. Compassion is an appreciation that suffering and illness engender special needs for comfort and help without evoking excessive emotional involvement which could undermine professional responsibility for the patient.

I would add loyalty to that list.

12

How Can the Placebo Work?

The null hypothesis about the placebo is that it has no effect at all other than as a marker or pointer. That is, people are most likely to call their doctors when their symptoms are at their worst after they have endured them as long as possible. Since most problems go away, especially the 80 percent of complaints for which patients seek medical help and which have no "structural" basis, then the placebo may simply be given credit for the natural history of disease. If the patient has called at about the time that the disease was about to improve on its own, then the doctor or the placebo may well get the credit. This is, I agree, a problem that makes evaluation of so many contentious claims difficult. The foregoing chapters have largely suggested that it is complaints rather than diseases which are improved and so in the rest of this chapter, I will look at the *potential* mechanisms by which pain can be assuaged. We are considering acute changes, even if it is difficult to decide exactly what we mean by "acute" given the wide ranges of phenomena claimed to be changed by placebo administration. James had the same problem when he writes about physical changes which "follow at some *remote period* because the mental state was once there."[1] Let me emphasize that the explanations I will consider in what follows all have to do with relief of pain. To consider mechanisms by which blood pressure is lowered, for example, would lead me far afield.

At last we must ask, "How does the placebo work?" Or at least, "How do people think it works?" Theories abound, but none are proven. Some derive from observations in patients, and others from

---

1. James, W., *The principles of psychology*, New York: Dover, 1950.

animal experiments. I shall put observations in animals largely aside since by my definition, at least, the placebo response of humans cannot be studied in animals; investigators have no way of knowing how much animals contemplate or have faith in the future. I do not know whether the physiological effects of anticipation have been looked at in other than the Pavlovian mode. Yet it is surely not appropriate to compare the whole of the placebo effect in a human, even by inference, with whatever a dog feels when it wags its tail, salivates, or even modulates its immune responses.

A long tradition of behavioral science suggests that in animals placebo effects could be conditioned responses and that these same mechanisms can operate in humans, particularly those in chronic pain. Cardiovascular responses, mediated by the autonomic nervous system, can also be altered by operant behavioral techniques. Later in this chapter I will review some of the material as it applies to the placebo response. Even conditioning has been claimed to modify the immune response, both cell-mediated and humoral, in rats susceptible to the development of autoimmune disease. Receiving the gift of a pill from a physician may very well activate responses conditioned in the infant by loving relatives. Animal experiments help to suggest in part what happens in humans, but people are more than their behavioral responses.

In the context of placebo giving in clinical practice, the intent of the physician giving a symbol of help to the patient who is ready to accept it forms an integral prelude to the placebo effect. Placebos without such intent may bring benefit when the physician intends to deceive, even when only the patient has faith that a medication will work. Pain can even be relieved on the hospital wards when the resident physician gives saline to a hostile "old crock." That shows us the power of hope and faith. But respect for truth-telling, and concern for informed and educated patient equality, will no longer allow most physicians to use the placebo to deceive. That the placebo works even when it is used as a challenge from an adversary position deepens the mystery.

How does a placebo work? All theories so far implicitly if not always explicitly accept the idea that only pain perception changes; illness improves, but disease processes remain unaffected. There is much talk of dramatic improvement in disease, but miracle cures turn phantasmagoric under scrutiny. A few commentators discuss dramatic reports of cures, as seriously as theologians discussing transsubstantiation, but in their explanations they return to brain events only.

The mind-brain dichotomy figures strongly in all explorations of how the placebo works, but the domains of psychiatry which studies the mind and neurobiology which studies the brain are a long way from confederation. Those who hold to the brain as a machine-computer focus on mechanisms such as the neuroendocrine apparatus discussed in chapter 7. They see all mental disease or mental effects as biochemical in origin, depression, for example, being a derangement of catecholamine metabolism, or "hard-wired," fixed neural connections sprouting during fetal life and for sometime afterward in a way that makes the early environment permanently responsible for later behavior. Those who look on the mind as more than the sum of its fixed structural components look to what ideas stimulate the placebo response and talk about symbols, conditioning, and the like. No one has yet subjected the brain of someone getting a placebo to positron emission transmission studies, to watch the brain think, and so most explanations of the placebo response remain conjectural.

We do have to ask why some people, patients or subjects, respond to a placebo and others do not. Presumably everyone has the same neuroendocrine apparatus and the same ability to respond, and in the answer to that question—which I do not have—must come the explanation of why the placebo reaction characterizes about 35 percent of the population. Whether that 35 percent can be traced genetically and whether placebo responsiveness will some day be in the same category as color-blindness, or whether placebo responsiveness—which I prefer to believe—depends upon the development of specific ways of responding to certain stimuli, in fact a learned reaction, is of course difficult at present to discuss. Given the difficulties inherent in the mind-brain problems, I will deal with how a placebo works, or at least what the current theories are.

Most of those theories have to do with the mind-brain and have been divided (by Byerly,[2] and subsequently Brody,[3]) into (1) "mentalistic," having to do with a patient's state of awareness, and (2) "conditioning," changes in "outwardly observable behaviors." Under the former comes the engendering of transference, hope, and other constructive emotions, explanations which are beyond current display on video monitors, but which have to do with the patient's perception of pain. "Conditioning" encompasses observations about stimulus-response and learned behavior which are more congenial to post-Skinnerian observers. The mechanisms may be (1) physiologic and related to endorphin stimulation or to cortical influences on the gate mechanisms, (2) mental and the result of transference, or (3) psychologic and related to conditioning. Observers often comment on "the natural healing processes," but I have difficulty defining them though

2. Byerly, H., Explaining and exploiting placebo effects, *Persp. Biol. Med.* 19:425–36, 1976.

I recognize the tendency of the healthy body to try to repair itself. Any effect on the healing state is difficult to define with current knowledge, and, as much of the foregoing discussion in this book has suggested, there is little if any evidence that placebos affect more than pain and suffering.

Even if the placebo effect proved largely mentalistic, it would bring no less benefit. Reactions to physical illness, or the psychological reactions to feelings of vulnerability, are intensified by physical abnormalities and play a large role in the feelings of "illness."

BEHAVIORAL MECHANISMS

Behavioral mechanisms by which the placebo could have an effect have been suggested with enthusiasm: the expectation of the patient modulates the effect of drugs. Although they are similar, behavioral concepts involve simple experiments around the pill and more complex ones around the response of the subject.

The Effect of the Pill

For the first, the placebo effect is a very simple conditioned response: a pill is supposed to help, and the placebo brings relief at least partly because of its association with other more effective medicines that have been taken before. Much research has gone into the appropriate color, size, taste, and other attributes of the placebo stimulus. The material can be reviewed in detail in Jospe's *The Placebo Effect*.[4] These experiments take the subject as a kind of fixed response to stimulus and regard the pill's visual properties as more interesting. The concept seems analogous to a vending machine which drops out bottles of soda when the appropriately sized coins are inserted.

Central Excitation

A second explanation looks at richer behavioral mechanisms. Everyone knows what conditioning is all about, the increasingly firm response of a subject, animal or human, to a positive reception to that response. Behavior is sensitive to the consequences that it invokes and in a sense is therefore partially controlled by those consequences. If you laugh when I tell a joke, I will tell more; if you frown, I will stop. In the Pavlovian laboratory at Johns Hopkins University, investigators noted that an observer just watching conditioning trials to study

3. Brody, H., *Placebos and the philosophy of medicine*, Chicago: University of Chicago Press, 1980.

4. Jospe, M., *The placebo effect*, Lexington, MA: D. C. Heath, 1978.

heart rate had a marked effect on that heart rate.[5] A number of studies led to the conclusion that persons involved in the care of animals during the development of an abnormal heart rate could evoke that abnormal heart rate simply by appearing in the laboratory. The reaction was specific to the persons involved, as strangers did not evoke the same response, conclusions certainly the very apotheosis of Heisenberg's theory about the effect of an observer.

The Impact of the Doctor

Gleidman, Gantt, and Teitelbaum suggest that "The impact of the doctor on the patient can be such as to modify or worsen the disease, depending to some degree on the meanings the patient has learned about certain help giving situations in the past. To the extent that doctors and therapy have come to stand for relief of stress, the patient's response is likely to be favorable."

Placebo as Conditioned Response: Neuroimmunology

Based on their own explorations and on a literature review of largely animal research, Ader and Cohen have organized a fuller theoretical model of the placebo effect as conditioning.[6] Their proposals, which lie somewhere between the simple Pavlovian stimulus response and the central excitation of the Hopkins group, carry the implicit assumption that the higher levels of the human brain do not override lower connections enforced by the repeated association of neutral events with stimulated responses. That is, I can train my dog to fetch the newspaper by offering him a bone when he brings it back, and humans may well respond to the therapeutic situation by feeling better on getting any pill. Yet I cling to the hope that the physician-patient encounter, between two people, may be more, should be more, than a primitive conditioned response. To be sure, if there has been little talking and less listening, no reassurance or comfort or plan of action, then the physician-patient model may fulfill the criteria of a conditioned response. I must take the conditioning model to offer a partial, not a total, explanation of what happens when the patient takes an inactive pill which his physician has given him.

To return to Ader and Cohen's observations, repeated injections of amphetamine lead rats to increased motor activity, which then also oc-

5. Gleidman, L. H., Gantt, W. H., and Teitelbaum, H. A., Some implications of conditional reflex studies for placebo research, *Amer. J. Psychiatry* 113:1103–07, 1957.

6. Ader, R., and Cohen, N., Behaviorally conditioned immunosuppression, *Psychosomatic Med.* 37:333–40, 1975; Ader, R., Conditional immunopharmacologic effect in animals: Implication for a conditioning model of pharmaco therapy, in *Placebo: Theory, research, and mechanisms*, ed. L. White, B. Tursky, G. E. Schwartz, New York: Guilford Press, 1985.

curs after injections of simple saline, such a response to a "placebo" presumably being conditioned by the consequences of the amphetamine so that hyperactivity is associated with any injection. If an injection can become a conditioned stimulus for rats, they suggest that in humans the "entire ritual surrounding drug administration" can also be a conditioned stimulus.

Even immunological reactivity can be conditioned, to some extent, according to observations which have bolstered the new field of psychoneuroimmunology.[7] Ader and Cohen gave saccharin-flavored water to animals along with an immunosuppressive drug, expecting that the distinctive flavor of saccharin would be associated with the effect of the immunosuppressive agent as the unconditioned stimulus. Animals so conditioned to saccharin mounted a lesser immunological response to antigen than those who got saccharin and antigen, but in whom saccharin had not previously been linked with immunosuppressive drugs. In succeeding studies they have even shown that pairing saccharin with an immunosuppressive stimulus can make it possible for saccharin alone to suppress the graft-versus-host response; using an autoimmune disease model in mice they report that conditioned mice reexposed to "neutral" (nonimmunosuppressive) stimuli previously associated with immunosuppression develop the autoimmune disorder more slowly than unconditioned animals.

Such studies offer persuasive evidence that mental stimuli can affect the immune system. One problem, as Ader has recognized, however, is that the effects are small enough to require statistical manipulation for significance. Yet the evidence is impressive that the immune system is subject to some kind of modulation by the brain. In this they follow in a very long Rochester tradition which many years ago suggested that loss of a loved one preceded the onset of cancer in humans. The Simontons of Texas support this belief in their suggestions that depression inhibits the immune response; they ask their cancer patients to try to visualize the white cells and immunocytes destroying cancer cells, and they routinely refer cancer patients for psychological exploration to look for depression preceding the development of cancer.[8]

Ader and Cohen see such immunoregulation as an extension of drug-induced conditional physiological responses: they look on any drug regimen as a conditioning model that might be sensitive to manipulation. The pharmacophysiological effect elicited by a drug is the

7. Solomon, G. F., The emerging field of psychoimmunology, *Advances* 2:6–19, 1985.

8. Simonton, O., Matthews-Simonton, S., and Creighton, J., *Getting well again*, Los Angeles: Tarcher, 1978.

unconditioned response, the drug the unconditioned stimulus.[9] The environment (doctor's office) or behavioral events (reassurance by the physician) or stimuli (physician's white coat) are all associated with the drug that is given to become conditioned stimuli. Repeated pairing of a conditioned stimulus with an unconditioned stimulus ultimately allows the conditioned stimulus to elicit a response much like that previously evoked by the active drug. On this model, going to a physician makes you feel better simply because going to physicians has made you feel better before. Going to a doctor who gives you a pill, even if he tells you that the pill is inactive, makes you feel better willy-nilly because of your conditioned response. The explanation offers one reason why patients with obscure pains and weakness respond so well to injections, according to common if uncontrolled clinical observations. Vitamin B-12 injections sometimes relieve pain and weakness because they elicit a conditioned response in patients who have benefitted before.

It is important to keep in mind that some experimental evidence suggests that the conditioned response need not be in the same direction as the drug with which it was originally linked. Matters are more arcane than I can cover, but studies of morphine have suggested that *hyper*algesia may be the conditioned response rather than the expected analgesia.[10]

Looking at controlled trials, Ader sees the placebo effect as being simply the result of continuous reinforcement, at least for the group getting the active drug, whereas the controlled group gets no reinforcement because the drug that they are getting is "inactive." Ultimately, Ader suggests that a partial reinforcement schedule, giving placebo and drugs in varying proportions, might make it possible to reduce drug dosage, some side effects, and even the duration and cost of pharmacological therapy.

For Ader, "The therapeutic effect of a placebo is not something mystical, it is not a trick, and it is not a lie. As a bona fide learning phenomenon, the 'placebo effect' is amenable to experimental analysis and, rather than having been over-estimated, its potential therapeutic effects have probably been under estimated."[11] What they called the "central psychological state" was important to conditioning. They suggested that the doctor who induced a comparable state in the patient can "thereby make this patient receptive to the changes the doc-

9. Eikelbaum, R., and Stewart, J., Conditioning of drug-induced physiological responses, *Psychological Rev.* 89:507–28, 1982.

10. Ibid.

11. Ader, Conditional immunopharmacologic effect.

tor communicates as necessary for health." In animals a stimulus ineffective by itself proved effective when it was followed by feeding,
which they took to impose "central excitation": "In a sense, this may
be a paradigm of the therapeutic situation where changes towards
health are induced in the patient by a doctor who is able to cultivate a
basic state of arousal."

They look upon the doctor as a conditional signal and suggest that
patients may try to meet their doctor's expectations because of anticipated approval, respect, understanding, and so forth:

> If a patient is hospitalized and removed from the setting which
> produced or keeps his illness alive, this may lead to improvement
> regardless of the therapeutic procedures employed. Where place-
> bos were involved, the tendency would be to relate improvement to
> their use, although the change, more likely, may represent the
> diminution of symptoms as a result of the process of extinction.

For Skinner and his students pain behavior has become the "operant," that is, the response is potentially subject to voluntary control
and is subject to influence by consequences.

These suggestions, now over twenty years old, are pertinent not
only to general medicine but to the placebo. Giving a placebo may
evoke only a conditioned reflex, whether to the gift or to the physician is uncertain. But if the patient has had previous bad experiences
with physicians or with medications, the physician or the placebo may
provoke anxiety or other adverse reactions, leading to an ineffective
placebo or even to an adverse effect. It used to be accepted that some
physicians were "better healers" than others, but the idea that they
stimulate conditioned responses, as suggested by Skinner a few
years ago, has not received very much attention from the medical
profession.

Extinction—removal from a stimulus over a long period of time
—usually decreases a conditioned response. Reinforcement—returning the subject to the situation in which the responses were first
engendered—reactivates those responses. Relief of symptoms on admission to a hospital is the result of removing the patient from an
anxiety-provoking situation, which can be seen as a stimulus-response
situation.

Wellness Behavior

In general behavioral therapy aims at reinforcing wellness behavior rather than sickness behavior. This is easier to state than to understand, but in general, behavior modification aims at reinforcing responses which make a patient feel better rather than those which
make him feel worse. In the category of illnesses considered to com-

prise sickness behavior Miller lists "fatigue, weakness, various complaints, wincing, limiting physical activity, and other signs of pain."[12] In the behavioral mode the placebo presumably reinforces certain responses tending to wellness behavior and may help the patient to increase his feelings of competence and control. Appetite comes in eating. That suggestion is an important factor is hard to avoid.

MENTAL MECHANISMS

Symbolic Effects of Placebo

What kind of mental event stimulates the stipulated physiological mechanisms? Very little is known. Symbolic meanings have exerted a powerful attraction. The placebo is a symbol of the physician's power to heal, or I would say, to comfort, affecting solely the perception of pain. Important, too, may be that the pill is swallowed, becomes part of the patient, and for patients with digestive troubles that aspect of incorporation may be very important. More than a silent gift from physician to patient, the placebo is a symbol of beneficence.

Placebo as Symbol

Frank sees the placebo as a form of psychotherapy: "The administration of an inert medicine by a doctor to a patient is also a form of psychotherapy, since its effectiveness depends on its symbolization of the physician's healing function."[13]

For Flanders Dunbar, the right symbols by themselves had a healing aspect.[14] She emphasized the healing effect of rituals using symbols, and we can accept that idea. If the placebo is to function as a symbol, it has to be a culturally accepted, understood symbol. Giving a gift falls into that category. Receiving a medication from a physician is receiving a gift as a promise.

Psychoanalysts emphasize the symbolic effect of the placebo for the patient. For Krystal a placebo gives the patient the freedom to exercise certain adult functions; if I interpret him correctly, the placebo functions as a symbol of an external loved one, especially for "psychosomatic" and "drug dependent" persons: "The patient becomes able to exercise his hitherto inhibited functions, but he denies his part in it, and attributes the activity to the pill. The ingestion of the pill repre-

12. Miller, N. E., Behavioral medicine: Symbiosis between laboratory and clinic, *Ann. Rev. Psychol.* 34:1–31, 1983.
13. Frank, J. D., *Persuasion and healing*, New York: Schocken, 1970, p. 3.
14. Dunbar, F., *Psychiatry in the medical specialties*, New York: McGraw Hill, 1959.

sents a ritual or symbolic act through which one gains access to a function which otherwise remains blocked."[15]

Krystal suggests that the placebo, the biofeedback machine, the shaman's incantations, and the hypnotist's suggestions all work much the same, to help the patient exercise control of "previously inhibited" functions. In his view the placebo is simply a means to overcome an internal block.

James had his usual pertinent comment: "The medico-materialistic explanation is that simpler cerebral processes act more freely where they are left to act automatically."[16]

Symbol as Conditioned Stimulus

For some psychiatrists the placebo functions as a symbol which then exerts its beneficent effect. Neutral signals can serve as symbolic stresses. As Wolf suggests, "It is probable that most adaptive functions of the cardiovascular system are responsive to stimuli that owe their force to their special significance to the individual."[17]

As an example of this phenomenon, Lown told of a forty-year-old man with far-advanced coronary artery disease.[18] Enrolled in an exercise tolerance testing program, the patient "observed that he was compelled each time to stop precisely after 44 crossings of the two steps." To look for a conditioned reflex, Lown began to count aloud the number of times the patient had crossed the two step platform after he had gone more than halfway. At first Lown gave an honest count; as the patient got toward twenty-eight or so, he would call out, "twenty-nine," "thirty," and so forth. The patient consistently developed angina and electrocardiographic changes at the forty-fourth count. After a while Lown began deliberately to give a false count, when the patient reached twenty-eight crossings calling out "forty, forty-one, forty-two," and so forth. At each false count of forty-four the patient complained of chest pain and the electrocardiographic pattern showed changes identical to those of a longer period of exertion. When the patient became aware of the deception, he no longer developed pain until a true count of forty-four.

This experience suggested that calling out the sequence to forty-four became associated with pain and that the verbal clue, that is the count of forty-four, was responsible for the development of the pain.

15. Krystal, H., Self-representation and the capacity for self-care, *Annual of Psychoanalysis* 6:209–46, 1977.

16. James, W., *The varieties of religious experience*, New York: Modern Library, 1902.

17. Wolf, S., Cardiovascular reactions to symbolic stimuli, *Circulation* 18:287–92, 1958.

18. Lown, B., Verbal conditioning of angina pectoris during exercise testing, *Amer. J. Cardiol.* 40:630–34, 1977.

Such an excellent example of how symbols can affect pain perception—in Lown's case for the worse—must make us ask whether if a count of forty-four can be so powerful, what effect some of the words, comments, and attitudes of the physicians and other members of the healing professions evoke.

I wondered why Lown waited twenty years to write up this report; I conjectured that it might have been a change in his own perception, new confidence that the view of a respected elder statesman (and now Nobel prize winner) would not be derided, or a change in what is acceptable to editors and to the general medical public. In response to my inquiry, he wrote: "These experiences were so important in shaping my clinical outlook that I felt obliged to share them with colleagues. I have frequently related them in lectures. It has always been easier to present these observations to lay than to medical audiences, largely, I presume, because doctors have been miseducated and conditioned virtually to disregard biobehavorial factors. A pretentious 'scientism' mars the physicians' perception of the power of the placebo—be it word, pat, or pill."[19]

Symbol for Physician

But the placebo works in both directions as an icon to focus attention; it affects the physician as well as the patient. The placebo tells the patient that the physician is going to try to help, but just as important, it reminds the physician that there is a person, not just a disease, out there. I like to think that the placebo affects the physician as much as the patient, evoking in him a new state of mind, reminding him that medicine is more than mathematics. Giving a placebo whose mechanism is so baffling should remind the physician that he must be humble before his ignorance, that he is still but one person treating another.

Getting physicians to think more about persons would be a lot, even so. To many patients physicians have become remote impersonal figures. They talk to each other and to the patient only in an arcane code, a shorthand which mystifies and, some still believe, is designed to confuse. Modern technology is so precise that physicians should have more time to talk to their patients. Instead the images now so useful, echoes, CTs, and MRI evoke increased communication between physician and physician, but still short-circuit the patient. Giving a placebo in the proper spirit requires communication between physician and patient.

Physicians, of course, may have the same kinds of conflicts as patients, and may respond to the attitudes of their patients from their

19. Lown, B., personal communication June 6, 1985.

own neurotic needs: Havens has suggested that the patient who doesn't get better may threaten the doctor's sense of "narcissistic integrity." He reminds us that "contact with new patients and their families may revive the internist's strong feelings of strain or anxiety. Medical caretakers may react adversely when they are not loved or admired by their patients."[20] The doctor must respond to the patient from an equally realistic recognition of his own fears of therapeutic failure. Giving a placebo does away with confrontation and, by bringing about a mutual recognition of uncertainty and by bringing that uncertainty to a conscious level, may help to mobilize empathy and other presumably helpful emotions.

TRANSFERENCE

The importance of transference for the placebo effect in any "mentalistic" scheme is crucial. The emotional bond, born of inequality between patient and physician, of a real dependency of the patient on the physician, leads to an unrealistic overevaluation of the physician by the patient and to a transfer to the physician of emotions the patient once had, as a child, to other important authority figures. Analysts try to safeguard their patient's autonomy and indeed to strengthen it, but their goal is an understanding of the personality and its neuroses. Greenacre suggests, that "the chief safeguard is the analyst's sticking to the work of actually analyzing, and not serving as guide, model or teacher no matter how luring these roles may be."[21]

For the nonanalytic practitioner these other roles serve a helpful purpose. Most physicians take them on, some more easily than others. For a nonanalyst like me, the placebo seems to focus the transference reaction, somehow intensifies it by the act of giving and receiving, and facilitates that still mysterious transaction, the relief of pain. The placebo no doubt symbolizes the continuity of the patient-physician relationship. To be sure it might be argued that to have the patient rely on, even receive, such a "magical" mechanism diminishes his autonomy. That may well be, but the connection between one person and another is important in the relief of pain.

Psychoanalysts recognize that even in the "compensated adult" there are submerged attitudes and feelings about stress and helplessness which are reactivated and intensified by any illness.[22] To some

20. Havens, L., personal communication, Dec. 26, 1985.

21. Greenacre, P., The role of transference, *J. Amer. Psychiatr. Assoc.* 2:671–84, 1954.

22. Bibring, G., and Kahana, R., *Lectures in medical psychology*, New York: International University Press, 1968.

extent, they point out, such "regression" to a more infantile state can be helpful or harmful; the patient who readily assumes a passive-dependent role after an operation serves his own interest by doing what he is told. The patient who "needs to defend against these fears by inappropriate demonstrations of his strength and virility" may not cooperate with his postoperative treatment and hinder recovery.

That is not so very different from James's comments about the religion of healthy-mindedness:

> Under these circumstances the way to success, as vouched for by innumerable authentic personal narrations, is by an anti-moralistic method, by the "surrender" of which I spoke . . . passivity not activity; relaxation not intentness . . . Give up the feeling of responsibility, let go your hold, resign the care of your destiny to higher powers.
>
> The mind-curers have given the widest scope to this sort of experience. They have demonstrated that a form of regeneration by relaxing, by letting go, psychologically indistinguishable from the Lutheran justification by faith and the Wesleyan acceptance of free grace, is within the reach of persons who have no conviction of sin.[23]

In a sense in a secular age the placebo function is to focus, as I have suggested over and over again, on the relationship between patient and physician. In a religious age the same was achieved by rituals of another variety.

Could transference have a therapeutic effect of its own? Does accepting dependency, returning to a childlike state, the very act of being helped, have any physiological effect? This is the same question posed earlier about the physiological (and possibly beneficial) effects of emotions other than the aggressive ones. If transference is a customary normal human phenomenon, as its very ubiquity suggests, if transference stands for the contact of one human with another, then we certainly may ask whether such connections could bring physiologic or even therapeutic benefits beyond their importance in the psychoanalytic transaction.

Is it the transference which is helpful or is it the context of the analysis? That is, could transference alone be helpful without regard to the theory behind the therapy? As Brian Bird points out, there may be a direct *nonanalytical* helpfulness in the analytic situation which may be mistaken for help by the analysis.[24] Going to a doctor brings its

23. James, The varieties of religious experience, pp. 108, 109.

24. Bird, B., Notes on transference: Universal phenomenon and hardest part of analyses, *J. Amer. Psych. Assoc.* 20:267–300, 1972.

own placebo effect; the very act of going to an analyst, deciding to undergo psychoanalysis, may, in itself, be helpful aside from the specific content of the analysis. That in large part is the message from the controlled clinical trials of various drugs. The same questions are being asked about psychoanalysis at present.

Countertransference

Giving a placebo symbolizes direct support of immediate problems. Transference, the readiness of the patient to relate unrealistically to the physician, has much to do with the process. Countertransference, the unrealistic assessment of the patient by the physician, must play a role in enhancing the ability of physician and patient to work together, to alert the internal power of the patient. The placebo may mobilize the healing power of the patient, but it also gives the all too human physician time to focus on the patient, to act as a symbol for the patient.

SUGGESTION

The placebo, of course, may just enhance the therapeutic effect of suggestion, on which doctors used to rely so strongly.

James points out that " 'suggestion' is only another name for the power of ideas, *so far as they prove efficacious over belief and conduct*" (p. 110).

Lipkin draws the distinction between *persuasion*, the act of influencing by argument or reason, and *suggestion*, a process of impressing an idea or attitude upon the mind of another by intimation or insinuation. To some extent suggestion is less obviously rational than persuasion.[25]

Paul Kaunitz, a professor of psychiatry at Yale, comments on why he offers most patients a favorable prognosis: "positive reinforcement can foster optimism which in turn may offer the patient a more hopeful outlook and an inducement to become well." Of the therapist he states: "it is his responsibility to influence, to the best of his ability, the patient's psychological mechanisms and external environment, so that nature's forces can bring to the fore the individual's underlying strength."[26]

We return to faith, hope, and expectation in the power of suggestion. Going to an analyst and going to a healing shrine may have their parallels. Several studies disagree on whether psychotherapy of any

25. Lipkin, M., Suggestion and healing, *Perspectives Biol. Med.* 28:121–26, 1984.
26. Kaunitz, P., The favorable prognosis, *Conn. Med. J.* 49:543, 1985.

variety brings results superior to those of a placebo.[27] There are many difficulties inherent in assessing the results of psychotherapists in general; just as one physician is better at reading X-rays for reasons which have more to do with his ability to see than with his training, so others must be better at healing or comforting. I doubt that the questions about psychotherapy have been answered by studies so far, but they play upon the placebo, and the question of whether one physician may give a placebo with more charisma than another.

DYADIC BOND

We know that mental events affect physiology and, with Cousins, we can ask if gratitude or hope or other feelings have a physiologic effect. What is their influence on the much-credited endorphins? It has been suggested that the placebo symbolizes a "dyadic" bond, the relationship of one person to another, that somehow the placebo helps to locate the patient in relation to his physician, that it helps to form a "group system," something like Alcoholics Anonymous or est, or many of the other comings together of people in a common cause. Loyalty, being seized by a commitment, may have some pertinence here, but I will postpone that consideration to the next chapter.

The dyadic bond sounds not so very different from the mystic unions of Eastern religions or of the Christian mystics. Adler and Hammett have developed the idea for current times:

> Group-system hypothesis appears to have the advantage of parsimony and simplicity of application to fields as otherwise diverse as politics, religion, psychotherapy, and general practice. We can, for example, beneath a variety of different labels, discern the integrating force of the group system in Alcoholics Anonymous, Synanon, religious cults, faith-healing, zealous political movements, brain-washing and many forms of psychotherapy. Psychodynamic-insight, psychotherapies and therapeutic communities alike provide the patient with both substitute relationships and a systematized Weltanschauung.[28]

They see the patient being swept up in some kind of healing mode. The physiological effect of gratitude has not been studied, but that

27. Prioleau, L., Murdock, M., and Brody, N., An analysis of psychotherapy versus placebo studies, *Behavior Brain Sci.* 6:275–85, 1983; Prince, R. H., Psychotherapy as the manipulation of endogenous healing mechanisms: A transcultural survey, *Trans. Psychiatry Res. Rev.* 13:115–33, 1976.

28. Adler, H. M., and Hammett, V. O., The doctor–patient relationship revisited, *Ann. Intern. Med.* 78:595–98, 1973.

does not mean that it does not exist. Knowing that someone else is in contact, that one is being cared for, may bring healing or at least may stimulate its beginning. The question really is, can symbols have any physiologic effect on their own? Only for a person conscious and sensitive enough to grasp them, I assume. And they might be different for different people. It is their interpretation which counts. In psychologic terms the affectional states are as likely to have an influence on physiological processes as any other emotion.

The Placebo as Psychotherapy

What is the difference between a placebo as I describe it and psychotherapy? The psychotherapist is a trained socially sanctioned healer who tries to produce certain changes in his patient's emotional state, attitude, and behavior. The placebo changes the perception of pain but does little to change attitudes or personality. Placebos and psychotherapeutic words both provide symbols, but one is an icon and the other a sign pointing toward the resolution of disturbances. In a sense the placebo functions on the irrational side of the relationship, magically or intuitively, whereas psychotherapy tries to work on the more mature and rational side of the therapeutic alliance.

THE THERAPEUTIC ALLIANCE

We may not be sure how the placebo works, but we can be sure that it helps. Perhaps it is simplest to look at the placebo as a gift from the physician to the patient and as a symbol of the physician's willingness to *do* something. That may sound paternalistic, too philanthropic as May would put it, but the relationship between patient and physician does inevitably involve one helping the other in his sickness. The physician has already asked the patient to give up his body, to look at it — as Spicker sees it — as the body that he *has*, not as the body that he *is*.[29] (I like Spicker's concept, but it may not hold for the new generation of college students who live *in* their bodies, but who are *not* really their bodies. They tune it up, exercise it, but the youngest generation seems to me to look on their own bodies as machines they possess, not bodies that they are). The patient has given up his autonomy and his privacy and in return the placebo comes as the symbol of the physician's willingness to give of himself, to give something. As Newton has put it, "I must know that the physician is in league with me against the sickness, not the other way around, or I would not consult him, and I can verify this alliance at any point during the course of treatment simply with a few minutes' conversation."[30]

29. Spicker, S. F., Terra firma and infirma species, *J. Med. Phil.* 1:104–35, 1976.
30. Newton, L., The healing of the person, *Conn. Med. J.*, 41:641–46, 1977.

Newton emphasizes the importance of the alliance between physician and patient against the disease and how crucial, vital even, is the patient's perception of that alliance. The placebo can be the symbol of that alliance. I like to suggest that the exchange which must go on between patient and physician for full alliance can be symbolized literally by the placebo, the gift. To be binding legally a contract must involve an exchange. The placebo, like any other pill, symbolizes that exchange.

Eisenberg has suggested how much less likely are depressive symptoms in someone with dependable friendships.[31] He was impressed by a study which showed that such complaints as tiredness, anxiety, depression, irritability, backache, headache, palpitations, dizziness, and breathlessness were less likely to be found in subjects with a confidant, or acquaintances in their neighborhood and at work. Although the study was not statistically significant, the trends were impressive to him: "That social bonding increases host resistance adds further support to the concept that the social environment is an important determinant of health status."

To be sure, longstanding depression may lead to isolation and could be its cause rather than its effect, but social bonds must influence symptoms. It may well be that the placebo simply symbolizes friendship and a connection even if only with the physician as friend. Consolation, after all, must have some connection with healing. No matter what else he does, the physician must enlist, incite, or excite the healing powers within, whatever the mechanism of such powers may be.

It should be clear that such considerations apply only to the relief of pain, suffering, or anguish. It would be going much too far to suggest that laying on of hands has ever been shown to cure structural disease.

There are many such studies, sometimes wrenched out of context or selected like the stepping stones across the river, but they are suggestive. At the Health Insurance Plan of New York patients who were "socially isolated and with a high degree of life stress" were four more times likely to die after a heart attack over the next three years than were those who had low levels of stress and isolation. The authors of this study suggested that a physiological mechanism, the catecholamines stimulated by stress, evoked arrhythmias.[32]

In the *New York Times* of September 18, 1984, an article called "Confiding in Others Improves Health", suggested that sharing one's

31. Eisenberg, L., A friend, not an apple, a day will help keep the doctor away, *Amer. J. Med.* 66:551-53, 1979.

32. Ruberman, W., Weinblatt, E., Goldberg, J. D., et al., Psychosocial influences on mortality after myocardial infarction, *NEJM* 311:552–59, 1984.

troubled feelings, even writing about them, made people less vulnerable to physical illnesses. This of course is abundantly clear to many psychotherapists and family physicians and lies at the basis of the confessional. James Pennebaker, a psychologist at Southern Methodist University, suggests that confiding in someone else protects the body against damaging internal stresses. People who are less able to share intimacies than others have less effective immune systems than some. Dr. Pennebaker contacted surviving spouses of people who had died suddenly, by suicide or automobile accidents, and he found that the survivors who had kept their grief to themselves had more health problems that those who talked over their grief with someone else.

Quoted in the same article at Harvard David McLelland found that people under stress who tried to suppress their problems had less effective immune systems than those who did not. In many ways this simply gives quantitative background to the old notion that the "sorrow which has no vent in tears makes other organs weep." We need to talk about our troubles to get relief and release. Further, it turns out that people in psychotherapy tend to consult physicians for medical problems less often than those not in therapy. Clearly when one confides in a spouse or a friend, one continually has to think of the other person's feelings and reactions, but that is not the case with a therapist.

A physician may help even more than a friend.

13

The Patient–Physician Relationship: Loyalty as Guide

I suggest here that loyalty is the best guide for the physician–patient relationship, although loyalty is not a term much favored in the 1980s. Loyalty provides the context in which the placebo should be given. Giving a placebo will not in itself change the quality of the physician–patient relationship, but thinking about what he is doing will at least make the physician stop to consider whom he is treating. To be sure the placebo can be given in many different moods and modes and all may prove effective, but loyalty provides one constructive framework from which to view the placebo. In writing about loyalty and its relation to medical practice, I may be appealing to antique abstractions, professional virtues that have no meaning to current physicians and that could seem to be the self-justification of an aging consultant. Yet recognizing that in linking loyalty and the placebo I run the risk of glorifying paternalism, patient dependency, and the spiritual arrogance of the physician, I see that relationship as one possible lesson from looking at the placebo. There are doubtless many others.

Loyalty suggests that it is not by our person alone that we are faithful, but by our profession and by our specific promise. Fidelity, on the other hand, implies a bond between persons which is not what the relationship between doctor and patient is all about. The *OED*, however, lists loyalty and fidelity almost as synonyms. *Fidelity* is "the quality of being faithful; faithfulness, loyalty, unswerving allegiance to a person, party, bond," while *loyalty* is "faithful adherence to one's promise, oath, word of honour." Still, I like the implications of *loyalty* because it suggests a professional rather than a personal bond, loyalty by virtue of our role and our promise, our oath really, than by our person. Fi-

227

delity to me is personal, loyalty is professional. Konvitz defines loyalty
as follows: "Loyalty is the virtue, state, or quality of being faithful to
one's commitments, duties, relations, associations, or values. . . . Anyone or anything to which one's heart can become attached or devoted."[1] The point is that loyalty need not be associated with patrio-
tism and political allegiance alone. Look briefly at what the medical
profession has had to say about its own obligation, as embodied in the
Hippocratic oath, printed in full below.

Oath

I swear by Apollo Physician and Asclepius and Hygieia and
Panaceia and all the gods and goddesses, making them my witnesses, that I will fulfil according to my ability and judgment this
oath and this covenant:

To hold him who has taught me this art as equal to my parents
and to live my life in partnership with him, and if he is in need of
money to give him a share of mine, and to regard his offspring as
equal to my brothers in male lineage and to teach them this art—if
they desire to learn it—without fee and covenant; to give a share of
precepts and oral instruction and all the other learning to my sons
and to the sons of him who has instructed me and to pupils who
have signed the covenant and have taken an oath according to the
medical law, but to no one else.

I will apply dietetic measures for the benefit of the sick according to my ability and judgment; I will keep them from harm and
injustice.

I will neither give a deadly drug to anybody if asked for it, nor
will I make a suggestion to this effect. Similarly I will not give to a
woman an abortive remedy. In purity and holiness I will guard my
life and my art.

I will not use the knife, not even on sufferers from stone, but
will withdraw in favor of such men as are engaged in this work.

Whatever houses I may visit, I will come for the benefit of the
sick, remaining free of all intentional injustice, of all mischief and
in particular of sexual relations with both female and male persons,
be they free or slaves.

What I may see or hear in the course of the treatment or even
outside of the treatment in regard to the life of men, which on no
account one must spread abroad, I will keep to myself holding such
things shameful to be spoken about.

If I fulfill this oath and do not violate it, may it be granted to me

1. Konvitz, M. R., Loyalty, in *Dictionary of the History of Ideas*, ed. R. P. Wiener, New
York: Scribner, 1973, pp. 108–16.

to enjoy life and art, being honored with fame among all men for all time to come; if I transgress it and swear falsely, may the opposite of all this be my lot.[2]

For physicians, the Hippocratic oath has come to symbolize their professional loyalty to their patients. Many medical schools have their graduating class recite that oath in the presence of parents, spouses, and friends, often along with the oath of Maimonides. The Hippocratic oath, unexamined and extolled, has stood for the physicians' highest view of himself and his professional activity.

Edelstein wrote in 1943: "As time went on, the Hippocratic Oath became the nucleus of all medical ethics. In all countries, in all epochs in which monotheism, in its purely religious or in its more secularized form, was the accepted creed, the Hippocratic Oath was applauded as the embodiment of truth."[3]

Castiglione, a physician and historian, said of "this precious document" that "this oath shows to what ethical heights the concept of professional practice had reached even in the times of the early medical schools of Greece."[4]

As it is not my purpose to review the history of the Hippocratic oath, let us turn from such self-congratulatory, though justifiable, encomia to some modern but idiosyncratic criticism. It is chastening for the physician to contemplate the downfall of the Hippocratic oath in the 1980s. Many medical students, regarding it as sexist and too authoritarian, refuse to repeat it even as a meaningless rite of passage. A leading critic of professional medical ethics, Veatch, rather disdainfully lumps the Hippocratic oath with other professional codes of ethics, to question "the authority of a professional group to set its own ethical standards."[5] He sees the Hippocratic oath and its pledge of loyalty "to the cult group" as a gratuitous promise which the new member makes on the assumption of a professional role.

Veatch complains that (1) physicians arbitrarily assume a role which affects other people who are not members of their profession, and (2) those affected by the physician's promise have not necessarily been asked whether they wish to be so affected. He grants that a physician may have special role-related duties and rights, possibly as a mandate from society, but he emphasizes that the codes of professional ethics, "are not generated by the broader population which is

2. Edelstein, L., *The hippocratic oath: Text, translation and interpretation*, Baltimore: Johns Hopkins Univ. Press, 1943, p. 64.

3. Ibid.

4. Castiglione, A., *A History of Medicine*, trans. E. B. Krumbhaar, New York: Knopf, 1947, p. 155.

5. Veatch, R. M., *A theory of medical ethics*, New York: Basic, 1981.

affected by their content. They are not even grounded in philosophical or ethical thought accessible to the broader population. The Hippocratic Oath itself contains a pledge of secrecy" (p. 89).

Veatch finds problems with any code of ethics, even one released for public scrutiny, because it is essentially a "professionally generated document." He seems to be arguing for "informed consent" on a larger, societal scale. Following May, he argues that the code is a gratuitous rather than a reciprocal act, bestowed by the profession without discussion with those whom it is intended to benefit. Claiming that the Hippocratic tradition has never involved "pledges or promises made with or accepted by those outside the professional group," he objects to the fact that the oath is paternalistic and philanthropic. The physician promises he will do what he believes will best benefit the patient, but this is not a promise made to the patient, nor one negotiated with or reciprocated by the patient. Veatch objects that there is "in principle no common ground for ethical discussion with those outside the group" (p. 96), and he does not wish to leave "matters that really count" to the consensus of the professional group. He is uncomfortable with the claim that outsiders cannot know the ethics of the group even though they are affected by it and he suggests that the outsiders need not take such a claim seriously. I am unaware that physicians make such a claim. In his analysis Veatch may not be thinking of contemporary physicians who certainly court outsiders and sometimes seem to abdicate all their ethical decisions to ethicists like him.

This is not the place to discuss Veatch's somewhat crabbed analysis of physicians' motives. He underestimates society's long acquiescence in the physician–patient relationship which implicitly suggests that most nonphysicians have assented to the consensus of paternalism and beneficence, even if a contract has not been written. We would have to look at the history of physician–patient relationships and variations in other cultures to find whether a common structure runs through them all. He overestimates the equality between sick patient and physician. The legalistic contract that he would set up to constrain patient and physician alike seems unworkable.

Such considerations will not hold us now. His views simply emphasize how far the Hippocratic oath has fallen, and how little professional loyalty means to those outside the profession. He concludes that "an ethic that professionals base on their own consensus of what their role entails has no ethical force, at least with non-professionals. It is doubtful such a standard can be called an ethic at all. It is really more a set of customs or mores governing behavior of members of a private group" (p. 107). He does not want unrequested loyalty, which brings mutual obligations like unrequested love.

THE PHYSICIAN–PATIENT COVENANT

The Religious Background

In analyzing the relationship between physician and patient, William May returns to the religious covenant between the Jews and God.[6] That included (1) "an original gift between the soon to be covenanted partners", the exodus from Egypt; (2) the promise based on that gift, the vows of the Jews at Mount Sinai; and (3) the acceptance of a ritual and moral obligation to which they would be faithful. For May the Hippocratic oath has three quasi-convenantal parts: (1) duties to patients; (2) obligations to teachers; and (3) the setting of both within the context of an oath to the gods. It is refreshing for physicians to have May take so much kinder an attitude toward the Hippocratic oath than Veatch.

May likes the word *covenant*, which for him "conveniently describes the distinctive obligations to one's teacher. Physicians undertake duties to their patients, but they *owe something* to their teachers. They have received goods and services for which they owe their filial services. Toward their patients, they function as benefactors, but toward their teachers, they relate as beneficiaries. This responsiveness to gift characterizes a covenant" (p. 110).

May sees referrals between physicians, their teaching activities, consultations and daily collaboration all strengthening the bonds between physicians. Their loyalty to each other grows as a response to gifts received and anticipated. On the other hand, as he analyzes matters, medical codes do not interpret duties to patients in the same way as a "partly responsive act for gifts and services received." He joins Veatch in seeing the relationship physicians confer upon patients by their own code as the "ultimately pretentious ideal of philanthropy, . . . "a wholly gratuitous rather than a responsive act" (p. 112). He reemphasizes how large a debt the physician owes the community for his education and other social largesse. Moreover, as he sees so acutely, a doctor cannot function without a patient: "No one can watch a physician nervously approach retirement without realizing how much the physician has needed the patients to be himself or herself."

Ultimately then, May suggests that a covenant in the original religious model is the best model for the physician–patient relationship. Such a covenant (he makes me almost want to capitalize the word) is more than a commercial contract, he claims. A contract, he agrees, at

6. May, W. F., *The physician's covenant: Images of the healer in medical ethics*, Philadelphia: Westminster, 1983.

least breaks with a more authoritarian model of parent or priest. It emphasizes informed consent rather than blind trust, and it acknowledges the symmetrical relationship between doctor and patient, the exchange of information for goods, services for money received. A contract also provides for legal enforcement and does not rely on charity, but simply hardens the deal made by two people in their own best interest, as they see it.

May does not like the contract model. He wants more and cannot get completely away from the gift relationship. The physician who gets up in the middle of the night because his patient has been admitted to the coronary care unit of the local hospital, who goes in to give support and to be there, even though he knows that the resident staff will care for the patient without him, surely cannot be responding simply for the extra fee that he will get. There must be more than self-interest, although the cynic will maintain that the doctor comes in at night to maintain control. Contract suppresses the element of gift. May admits that gift does play a role in medical practice: "I do not object to the notion of gift, but to the moral pretension of professionals who see themselves as givers alone." I think he wants the doctors to admit that they like getting paid.

May worries, correctly, that the contractual approach will limit the transaction between physician and patient, making for specified services for established fees and leaving no room for emergencies and contingencies. He wants the difference between a contract and covenant to be a difference in spirit rather than a difference in agreement and in exchange. As he puts it, covenants are internal, contracts are external. For him the Covenant has its background clearly rooted in the Old Testament flowering into the Christian setting: "The covenant in Christ, in effect, locates the self, the beleaguered fearful self, within the dynamic giving and receiving gift love and need love" (p. 127).

For May the ultimate solution then is found in what he calls fidelity. He tells us that "a cautiously wise medieval physician [whom he does not name] once advised his colleagues, 'Promise only fidelity!' " (p. 143). In the modern secular society of physicians comprised of many backgrounds—at least in the United States—grounding ethics in the "transcendental" (p. 130) may not serve, however comforting the notion may be. Covenant carries a religious historical connotation while fidelity brings with it the notion of faith. For such reasons, I prefer the term loyalty.

LOYALTY

Loyalty could provide a useful guiding principle for the relationship of professional to client, loyalty to what physician and patient agree should be the patient's best interests. The concept of loyalty has not received much attention over the past few decades largely, I suppose, because of the evils that loyalty to authoritarian rulers has brought. Although it is no longer fashionable to talk of duty or obligation, loyalty might still provide a useful guideline for most professionals in their relationship to clients. For the physician loyalty to the patient would mean supporting what physician and patient beforehand have agreed to be the patient's best interests. This need not call for a legalistic contract spelling out every move of the physician, but it certainly should lead to discussion and consideration of the role of the physician in the patient's life and death. Currently, living wills and durable power of attorney imply a need to protect the patients against the power of the doctors. I do not argue against such restraints, but only that reexamination of loyalty might help to make some of them unnecessary.

Royce's *The Philosophy of Loyalty* has a Victorian ring to those who have lived through the era of the concentration camps.[7] We might view untrammeled loyalty as dangerous, in a way that Royce might not have envisioned. Moreover, the current generation of physicians may be wary of so broad an abstraction, of so strong a commitment.

Royce defines loyalty as

> mean[ing], according to this preliminary definition: The willing and practical and thorough-going devotion of a person to a cause. A man is loyal when, first, he has some cause to which he is loyal; when, secondly, he willingly and thoroughly devotes himself to this cause; and when, thirdly, he expresses his devotion in some sustained and practical way, by acting steadily in the service of his cause. (p. 16)

While it is disconcerting for a modern American reader to find Japanese bushido, the code of the samurai, praised, and while Royce's idealism has a mid-Victorian transcendentalism to it, Royce's analysis of loyalty deserves reading by modern professionals.

In his lecture "Loyalty to Loyalty" he considers the causes which are worthy of loyalty. The patriot, the knight, the Japanese samurai all exemplify loyalty, but loyalty is more than the martial virtues. The captain of a ship is loyal too, but loyalty is more than the captain going

7. Royce, J., *The philosophy of loyalty*, New York: MacMillan, 1928.

down with his sinking ship. Royce suggests that soldier and captain are simply fulfilling their duty by established and customary routines. The loyal man can be loyal by some act "which no mere routine predetermines." He chooses as an example the behavior of the Speaker of the House of Commons when King Charles I came to arrest some of its members. The King asked the speaker whether he saw the wanted men in the House. Royce approves the Speaker's response: "The Speaker at once fell on his knee before the King and said: 'Your Majesty, I am the Speaker of this House, and, being such, I have neither eyes to see, nor tongue to speak save as this House shall command; and I humbly beg your Majesty's pardon if this is the only answer that I can give to your Majesty'." For Royce the Speaker had completely identified himself with his cause and had expressed himself as the servant of that cause. Royce suggests that loyalty means being the reasonable *willing* devoted instrument of a cause; or, I would add, of a person. He discusses loyalty to friends, to family, to gangs and nations, and finds that for true loyalty there has to be a free or autonomous choice. For Royce loyalty is not forced; there is always an element of free choice. The physician will recognize that free choice can change. Relationships change, people and patients do not remain the same always, and taking on loyalty to a patient does not mean that the relationship is for once and forever.

Loyalties will come into conflict and lead to destructive conflict. The more people that are bound up into a loyalty, the more a supreme good is attained. The more that loyalty is pitted against loyalty, the worse things are. He wants causes that will attract the loyalty of the most people.

I do not intend to examine Royce's philosophical reflections, but simply to emphasize his point that "loyalty, as we have defined it, is the willing devotion of a self to a cause. . . . The higher types of loyalty involve autonomous choice. The cause that is to appeal to me at all must indeed have some elemental fascination for me. It must stir me, arouse me, please me, and in the end possess me. . . . My loyalty never is my mere fate, but is always also my choice."

Loyalty requires an idea of community, as John Smith, one of the few modern students of Royce, explains.[8] The community supplies the grounds for the validity of logical principles. We physicians can abstract them from their connection with the church. Smith emphasizes how Royce maintained that scientific knowledge was never possible apart from a community with an ideal of truth to which the members of that community are devoted. The definition of science

8. Smith, J. C., *Royce's social infinite: The community of interpretation*, Hamden, CT: Anchor, 1969.

adopted early in this book requires observation, evidence, and validation for something to be accepted as "fact." Royce calls that a "community of interpretation." As Smith puts it, "Truth is a reality only in so far as the goal of this community is a reality, and the whole company of seekers for truth have worked in the belief, explicit or implicit, that such a goal is real." (p. 5). As Smith explicates Royce's notions, a community is not simply a "collection of individuals, but rather a unity which endures; . . . communities tend to be organized into more inclusive communities embracing greater numbers of members" (p. 131). The community for Royce provides the ultimate values of devotion which for Royce constituted his moral fulfillment.

That idea of community, which it is not my purpose to explore here in all its fullness, does, however, impell a nostalgic backward glance at the former community of physicians with their rules, obligations, set conduct, and loyalty to the profession as a whole as well as to each other. Maybe it was only in their writings, maybe only in the eyes of their acolytes. That community may have been a narrow one, concerned with etiquette more than ethics, but it provided some bounds for professional and even personal behavior. In a sense the training period for physicians brought into their mind and habits notions that they were joining a community. Maybe that community was self-seeking and to a critic might look like a benevolent parent–teachers association, but there was something in it for patients as well as for physicians. Today clinical activity is dominated by commercialism and competition, and medical practice is being pursued in the corporate spirit. Paradoxically, as practicing doctors unite in groups to work for ever-larger corporations, the notion of the medical profession as a calling, a community of people, appears dead, or at least naive. Something must be lost, for patients as well as physicians, when that happens.

Yet the community of science, the community of scholars in medicine, endures and grows. The active societies of scientists are loyal to the pursuit of truth. They may waiver in hiding error or not always searching it out aggressively enough and they often defend too rigorously the failings of one of their own. Yet in Royce's terms scientists represent a true community which uplifts and sustains itself in a way which practicing physicians no longer have available to them. There may be arrogance, ambition, craze for unlimited power and adoration among the scientists, but in their work and in their hearts—to one like myself now a nostalgic outsider—they look like a community. Maybe that is why such clinical organizations as the American Gastroenterological Association made up largely of practicing physicians uphold the scientific ideal. Science gives us our only vision of the absolute, binding physicians together in a notion that in fact they do make up a community. I have earlier reflected on the dangers of thinking that there is only one way, but a sense of community is what medical practitioners lacks at present, as the spirit of competition is fostered in economic programs to cut costs of medical care. That old clinical community might have been isolated and never quite the "beloved community" which Royce ultimately had in mind, but it provided a link between physicians that could not have been all bad.

What better cause for loyalty than the care of the patient? That union of passion, social utility, and intellectual interest fulfills all of Royce's criteria when he asks, "Is there a practical way of serving the universal human cause of loyalty to loyalty?" Physicians can answer yes to that question. More than humanitarians trying to help mankind as a whole, physicians are taking care of the persons before them. They have a definite personal special cause, their patients. Royce says:

> If I am to be loyal, my cause must from moment to moment fascinate me, awaken my muscular vigor, stir me with some eagerness for work, even if this be painful work. I cannot be loyal to barren abstractions. I can only be loyal to what my life can interpret in bodily deeds. . . .
>
> I shall serve causes such as my natural temperament and my social opportunities suggest to me. I shall choose friends whom I like. My family, my community, my country, will be served partly because I find interesting to be loyal to them.

Surely that could be a physician speaking. When Royce adds that loyalty affects fellow servants, the medical institutions come into view. He says, "All those duties which we have learned to recognize as the fundamental duties of the civilized man, the duties that every man owes to every man, are to be rightly interpreted as special instances of loyalty to loyalty."

Royce's prescription calls for emotion to be involved in loyalty, whereas the ideal of the physician–patient relationship has been more dispassionate, empathy, not sympathy. The emotion of the physician should be for his profession (dare I name it "calling?") and not for his patient. Moreover placebos can be given without commitment or emotion and still bring relief.

To some extent, of course, the notion of loyalty in medicine could repolish the old military metaphor which Winslow has derided as obedience to higher ranks and maintenance of confidence in authority figures. Winslow reminds us that the notion of medicine as war, now so persuasive, was particularly appropriate for nursing which had its beginnings with the work of Florence Nightingale during the Crimean War.[9] Loyalty was the virtue for the nurse: "Loyalty will I endeavor to aid the physician in his work," and as Winslow interprets outmoded loyalty, it meant refusal to criticize the hospital, training school, fellow nurses, or the physician under whom the nurse worked. I prefer to believe that to the physician loyalty means faithfulness to the patient.

Loyalty to the patient means many things. It raises questions about corporate practice of medicine, now so popular. It brings in to focus the conflicting obligations of the salaried physician to those who hire him and to those whom he treats. It even raises questions about who should enlist patients in controlled clinical trials. Such trials are essential for the assessment of clinical prospects, but I must wonder whether the physician who is "in charge" of the patient can put knowledge to be gained ahead of his patient's welfare unless he is convinced that the treatments to be compared are equal and that to trust to chance is not harmful. Loyalty to the patient will not permit the extra diagnostic test for a fee or the ordering of a study for defensive medicine. Thoroughgoing loyalty puts the patient's interest above all others, requires a second opinion in uncertainty, puts the patient's case above the physician's.

Loyalty and Promise

A promise is defined by the *OED* as "a declaration or assurance made to another person with respect to the future, stating that one will do, or refrain from, some specific act, or that one will give or bestow some specified thing." Lawyers look at a promise almost panegyrically, possibly because people breaking promises keep them busy. For lawyers, as Fried puts it, "the promise principle, . . . is that principle by which persons may impose on themselves obligations where none existed before."[10] Lawyers have written paeans to the contract and to promise as the medium by which civilized human beings exercise their liberties. A contract is the self-imposed obligation, "the will binding itself," and contracts exist to enforce promises. Legal contracts have three parts, promise, acceptance of that promise, and a consideration given for the promise. That consideration has to be palpable, actual, although it may be a counterpromise, "If you do X, I will do Y."

To make a promise is to state your intentions in a truthful way so

9. Winslow, G. R., From loyalty to advocacy: A new metaphor for nursing, *Hastings Center Report*, June 84:32–39, 1984.

10. Fried, C., *Contract as promise: A theory of contractual obligation*, Cambridge: Harvard University Press, 1981.

that the other person will rely on your promise, will trust in the future *actions* of the person making the promise, not merely—as Fried points out—in your "present sincerity." A promise commits the person who makes the promise to a future performance. It is self-imposed and in that sense differs from what Rawls calls "natural duties,"[11] which are obligations applying to and owed to anyone without regard to voluntary acts and with no necessary connection with institutions or social practices. For Rawls obligations that arise as the result of a voluntary act, specifically a promise, are normally owed to specific persons: "We assume obligation when we marry as well as when we accept positions of judicial, administrative, or other authority. We acquire obligation by promising." He emphasizes that a standard reason for making promises is to set up or stabilize a small scale scheme of cooperation or a particular pattern of transaction (p. 346).

The physician–patient encounter seems to fit that transaction. The physician implicitly if not explicitly says to the patient, "If you pay me money, I will look out for your interests. I will do the best that I can for you." The promise should be more than the commercial contract, but at least it should be as much. Loyalty comes into that promise. As Fried sees it, "the faithful carrying out of mutual promises that the parties, having come to understand their *separate* purposes, chose to exchange." They require a background, even if unexpressed, of shared purposes, experiences, "and even a shared theory of the world." For physicians the current commercial metaphor leaves loyalty out of contract and substitutes a dry legalistic relationship. Physicians are bound only to what they have committed themselves to do, not to a loyalty to loyalty.

I find the idea of promise, of taking on and stating an obligation, to be the promise of the placebo. One does not give a gift to anything but a person. (When we give a gift to a pet, it is giving a gift to the person we want it to be). Giving a placebo as a gift is, or should be, giving a symbol of a promise. That promise is what placebo represents. The physician tells the patient to rely not only on his present sincerity, but on his future performance. The self-imposed obligation, for payment received, is the physician's promise of loyalty to the patient. Such an idea might seem to enshrine a physician–patient relationship based on private practice only, but that is far from my mind. The relationship, however, is closest to a contract. Not a lawyer, I keep far from the more complex issues of third party contracts and other more sophisticated notions appropriate to modern medical arrangements.

Paradoxically, of course, at first glance the person making the promise also gives a gift if he prescribes a placebo. But I am suggest-

11. Rawls, J., *A theory of justice*, Cambridge: Belknap, 1971.

ing that the promise is symbolized in the placebo and that the consideration given by the patient is two-fold. On the one hand the fee sets up a continuing relationship between physician and patient. On the other, by turning over his body and his trust to the physician, the patient gives a second "consideration." That should further suggest a counterpromise, that the patient will be loyal to the physician. By this I mean that if the patient disagrees with what the physician suggests or if it is his intention not to work with the physician, that he will say so. Patients have duties and obligations which it is not my purpose to discuss now, but which deserve more attention.

Finally, of course, I cannot suggest that the promise by the physician is the promise of a specific act. Promises for specific acts or results very surely lead to law suits, based on the doctrine of *reliance*, a loss incurred without gain to the other, or more likely in medical practice on *expectation*, claims for the value of the expectancy that the promise created.[12] That is, if a plastic surgeon promises to remake an ugly man in the image of a movie star, and the patient ends up looking like a comedian rather than a "matinee idol," then specific expectancy damages might be created. The promise is to a mode of action, a loyalty to loyalty, as the patient and the physician come to agree on the interests of the patient.

Loyalty and the Placebo

Giving a placebo can be the first step in attesting to loyalty, but it should not be a substitute for the time and energy required for the "thorough-going devotion" of loyalty. A pill or a placebo may not be necessary, most of the time will not be required if the physician is aware of, and confident in, his own therapeutic powers.

In an era when physicians were more certain of themselves, Harold Wolff could say, "The giving of a pill by the physician to the patient is the symbol for the statement, 'I will take care of you.' "[13] But giving a placebo should have as great an effect on the physician as on the patient. When he prescribes a placebo, he should take on the obligation of loyalty. "Thorough-going devotion" to the patient's cause would permit the placebo as a beneficent act, not intended to fool, mystify, or demean, but simply as a way to help. The loyal physician can give a placebo as a gift, maybe even without any more explanation than, "I think this will help you", if he keeps the interest of his patient uppermost in his mind. Paternalistic? Maybe, but no more so than the reli-

12. Dawson, J. P., Harvey, W. B., and Henderson, S. D., *Contracts*, Mineola, NY: Foundation Press, 1982.

13. Wolff, H. G., DuBois, F., Gold, H., Cornell Conferences on Therapy: Use of placebos in therapy, *New York J. Med.* 46:1718–27, 1946.

able plumber who tells me to buy a new sink. Let me reemphasize that giving a placebo does not bring loyalty automatically. There is no transubtantiation here. Giving a placebo without a lot of consideration can glorify the physician's notion of himself as a magic healer, able to cure without thought and effort, and that is far from what I want to suggest.

14

Should the Placebo Be Used?

I

CONSOLATION AND SUGGESTION:
THE PROMISE OF THE PLACEBO

t is time to close. No philosopher, I have no final answers, no plan, no theory even, underpinned by logic. I simply have
recorded my reflections about trying to use placebos out of insight not
ignorance. For the placebo has proven my lens to look at the stresses
in medical practice, between *science*, what has to be measured and
tested, and *intuition*, the immediately apprehended, the unmeasurable. Medical knowledge depends upon science, but practice is both
science and art.

Magic and irrationality, of course, have no place in medical practice except as a spur to looking at forbidden questions. As science
opens the cell to discovery and provides keys to the cure of disease,
exploring some of the nonmeasuring aspects of medicine may tell us
much about ourselves. The certainty of the mystic is more absolute
than that of the scientist, though he cannot display it on a video monitor. Some day the billions of uncounted neurons in the human brain
may be traced out so that with a modem we can tape our patient's
thoughts and patch up his hope with enzymatic glues. But for the moment, and I think for centuries to come, mind and thought remain
more than hard- or soft-wired circuits. Science is curing disease, the
scientific method is the only way that advances in the material world
can be made, and I hope that nowhere in this book will anyone find
even the hint that I am antiscientific. But there remain at least for
now some matters that science cannot conquer. Medicine can be the
bridge between the two cultures.

The placebo relieves pain, but how is not yet known. Giving a placebo arouses behavioral or mental mechanisms which then turn on
physiological mechanisms of endorphins, neural circuits, and immu-

241

noneurology to let the neurobiological network relieve pain. The neural cleft may be the final common pathway, but a hierarchical system in which symbols excite behavioral mechanisms different for different people seems plausible. We cannot escape our bodies or our minds; our reflexes are conditioned, and transference is built into us. Symbols are our stimuli and each symbol carries its own message. The white coat stands for distance, sterility, and science. Placebos speak of concern, beneficence, and caring. They tell the patient that he has a doctor who knows that he cares for a person and reminds the doctor that, more than a body to examine and repair, he has a person to attend.

Suggestion must play an important role in the placebo effect, but it should come out of the therapeutic alliance of doctor and patient. Loyalty to the patient provides one unifying principle for the physician; the placebo stands for the promise to be loyal to the patient's best interests. But when physicians listen to their patients as closely as they now look at them, the placebo may prove only the symbol of a promise. When they listen to their patients for more than clues to disease, to the person who suffers, a placebo will no longer be necessary, because physicians will have learned once more that they can help some patients through themselves. The physician who gives a placebo should be saying implicitly to the patient, "I will be loyal to your interests and this is my promise." The placebo does not create loyalty; the physician must give it.

Words as Placebos

The placebo is powerless without the physician. But the effectiveness of specific medical therapy has made many physicians believe that they are only conduits of power, of pills and procedures, and that loyalty or fidelity are outmoded concepts of an era when physicians could only sit helpless at the bedside. Physicians need to regain confidence in the symbolic reality of medicine, to grasp once again that words can be placebos which help, and to regain confidence in talking to patients and even in giving advice and reassurance. Words must accompany therapy if illness is to be helped. Words can also be placebos.

In *The Therapy of the Word in Classical Antiquity*, Entralgo carefully if exuberantly traced the power of the word from Homer through Aristotle, to strengthen the concept of psychosomatic medicine.[1] Like Hippocrates, Entralgo does not take everything that the patient says to be correct. He advises the physician to listen to the patient, to investigate why the patient has symptoms, and only then offer an explana-

---

1. Entralgo, P. L., L. J. Rather and J. M. Sharp, eds. and trans., *The therapy of the word in classical antiquity*, New Haven: Yale University Press, 1970.

tion. Yet Entralgo traces how physicians since Hippocrates have mistrusted the psychotherapeutic approach, not from ill will but because they had nothing to measure. Since modern physicians want to confirm their observations by measurements, the sensations of the body, particularly the words which reflect and describe those sensations, have seemed much less reliable than objective findings. Ong, with his usual acute reflections on seeing and hearing, says that the "hypervisualism of science relies on reducing all sensations to visual."[2] But the vision for medicine is too distant. We have sacrificed intimacy for precision. And it is hard to talk to an icon.

Yet if words can exhort the healthy, can reassurance and comfort also mobilize "healing" in the sick? If putting thought into words distinguishes men from animals, the power of words should help the sick. As James put it, "An idea, to be suggestive, must come to the individual with the force of a revelation."[3]

Plato's comments, in book 4 of the *Laws*, are pertinent:

Then you also understand that sick people in the cities, slaves and free, are treated differently. The slaves are for the most part treated by slaves, who either go on rounds or remain at the dispensaries. None of these latter doctors gives or receives any account of each malady afflicting each domestic slave. Instead, he gives him orders on the basis of the opinions he has derived from experience. Claiming to know with precision, he gives his commands just like a headstrong tyrant. . . . The free doctor mostly cares for and looks after the maladies of free men. He investigates these from their beginning and according to nature, communing with the patient himself and his friends, and he both learns something himself from the invalids and, as much as he can, teaches the one who is sick. He doesn't give orders until he has in some sense persuaded; when he has on each occasion tamed the sick person with persuasion, he attempts to succeed in leading him back to health.[4]

Such persuasion or reassurance should, of course, not be indiscriminately given.

The ever-present need of people for some personal connection, for comforting words if not always for persuasion, has led to a growing interest in primary care and to the burgeoning of alternative healing practices, many of which we have seen as at least effectively placebic because they establish a connection. Physician and patient need

2. Ong., W. J., *Interfaces of the word*, Ithaca: Cornell University Press, 1977, chap 5, "I see what you say."

3. James, W., *The varieties of religious experience*, New York: Modern Library, 1902, p. 112.

4. Pangle, T. L., *The laws of Plato*. New York: Basic, 1980.

to understand each other better, to know where each stands on a number of medical issues. Being kept alive after incapacity, receiving chemotherapy, or giving away eyes or other organs after death are some important issues to talk about. How far to trace down each complaint might be equally fruitful to discuss. Of course most patients make that decision by going to a doctor only when they think they are really sick, but the strength of that stimulus varies enormously. How much information a patient wants can also be discussed. The physiology of my headache is unimportant if aspirin will take it away. If physician and patient agreed ahead of time that symptom relief made sense unless the doctor deemed the complaint a serious one, a great deal of expensive and useless effort might be saved. Too many non-medical observers fear that relieving pain by a placebo may hide a disease until too late. This betrays more faith in physicians than they have in themselves, or in placebos.

We need a rededication and a redirection of psychosomatic medicine, the idea that diseases are affected, even if not generated, by emotion, cultural, psychological events, the idea that the physician treats the whole person. Holistic medicine, shorn of its pretenses, is psychosomatic medicine. For even when there is organic disease, the patient's subjective response can be as important as any change in the disease itself. The patient with ulcerative colitis and rectal bleeding, poked, prodded, orifices penetrated, and given a prescription, may still worry about persistent bleeding. He may wonder whether his disease is getting worse, whether a cancer could have been missed, and what the future will bring. Urgent diarrhea may force a student to leave his classes; embarrassment may keep him from returning. A public officeholder may fear that the pressures of public life are making his disease worse and may abandon his career. The physician scrutinizing his sigmoid mucosa may be satisfied at the progress of the disease, but the patient is not.

There is no need to multiply examples, but simply to emphasize how much the patient brings to his disease. Yet modern training, which highlights the metaphor of physician as scientist or detective, makes it difficult for many physicians to feel comfortable or useful in the role of caretaker or reliever of symptoms. Suggest to a doctor that he first relieve indigestion with an H2 blocker without seeing an ulcer at endoscopy and he will be offended that you are not scientific. Suggest that he do it with an inactive pill and he will think you crazy!

Medicine, the Silent Art

The placebo then is a symbol of the doctor's loyalty, a promise to the patient, but a reminder to the doctor that medicine is more than science, that his art, his person, his dedication, are required. The placebo is only a convenient symbol for what the healer can do. A specific ministration which deserves respect, the placebo may not be as important as the person who gives it and the manner in which it is dispensed.

Virgil called medicine "the silent art."[5] The Hippocratic physicians of Greco-Roman time, fearful of the irrational ways of the Aesculapian priest-physicians, their chief competitors, abandoned songs and incantation, but also gave up the comforting words which had been the physician's stock in trade. The persuasive words of Homer's physicians had confronted human illness with prayer, magic charms, and cheering speech. Confusing persuasive words with incantations, physicians abandoned talking and persuading, which did not have any "real existence in scientific traditional medicine."[6] For a while, in the nineteenth and twentieth centuries, the spread of psychotherapy and psychosomatic medicine made it look as if physicians were beginning to talk to patients again, and to listen to them. Yet the imaging revolution in the 1970s and 1980s has pushed medical practice far toward the silent art once again. Medicine has become a world of silence between doctor and patient, broken by the beeps and whirrs of the monitors.

Not too long ago, I was chatting with a friend about one of his more perplexing patients. "I have done every study I could, and still I can't find any explanation for his abdominal pain," he lamented. The patient proved to be a resident physician on a large aggressive surgical service. When I asked whether my friend had also inquired into the patient's personal and emotional life, he laughed, "Howard, that's your idea. It's not mine." He wanted tests, not talk. In ignoring the personal life of his patient my friend was doing what he had been taught, to rule out detectable disease.

Western medicine for the most part has paid too little attention to the release of emotions, the cathartic effect of words. Catharsis for Aristotle was the effect, the emotional purgation, that a tragic poem or play has upon the whole person. Cousins's observations may be simply the other side of that long-standing tradition. Entralgo put it this way:

For Aristotle a physician who was able with his words to produce in a certain patient psychological effects similar to those of the tragic poem would be therapeutically more effective and complete than the one who sees therapeutic practice as only a "mute art," in the manner of the Vergilian Iapix. . . .

5. Entralgo, Ratler, and Sharp, *The therapy of the word.*
6. Ibid., p. 242.

Can it then be surprising that the word, an instrument so powerful and modifying in governing man's reality, should by itself, without the addition of a magical power, have the ability to achieve the
cure of human disease or at least to help in it?[7]

Hippocrates stated that "For some patients, though conscious that
their condition is perilous, recover their health simply through their
contentment with the goodness of the physician."[8] Surely emotions
are so invigorated by poetry, music, speech, plays, and movies that the
therapeutic power of words needs more attention and study. The
doctor who listens to his patient, who talks with them, may change the
direction, or at least the intensity, of their attention and so influence
their perception. An interpretation can be so helpful.

Jung suggested that

A psychoneurosis must be understood as the suffering of a human being who has not discovered what life means for him. . . .
The doctor who realizes this truth sees a territory opened before
him which he approaches with the greatest hesitation. He is now
confronted with the necessity of conveying to his patient the healing fiction, the meaning that quickens—for it is this that the patient longs for, over and above all that reason and science can give
him.[9]

Words which can have such powerful effects need not necessarily
come from a physician. The power of presidents, preachers, perform-
ers, and poets is a daily experience. Yet, Entralgo points out that not
only must the words be "beautiful and adequate," but

Only when the word comes from a man of prestige and is accom-
modated to the character and the mood of the hearer, only then
will it become fully efficacious. . . . Moreover, for the action of the
word to attain its greatest efficacy—and psychotherapeutic treatment especially demands this—it is necessary that the particular
relationship be established between the speaker and the hearer.

We may well ask whether a physician is necessary for such healing.
Must someone train through four years of college in molecular biology and the workings of the cell, then four years of medical school
and yet four more of residency and critical care medicine, to give
person-to-person healing? For practice in a hospital, to take care of

7. Ibid., pp. 242, 69.
8. Hippocrates, Precepts VI, in *Hippocrates*, W. H. S. Jones, trans., New York: G. P.
Putnam's Sons, 1923, p. 319.
9. Jung, C.: *Modern man in search of a soul*, New York: Harcourt, Brace, Jovanovich,
1933, p. 225.

diseases, such prolonged training is essential, to make the distinctions between illness and disease and to treat disease as well as illness. For office practice, to take care of most patients, a much wider background, as much in the humanities as in science, may well be in order. Only a physician trained in science can be trusted with a placebo.

No scientifically based physician could suggest that words—or any communication between physician and patient—affect more than the mind, more than the attitude and emotions of the hearer. Yet the interrelationships between the neuroendocrine apparatus of the brain and of the gut demand no great leap of faith to imagine that attitudes in the mind, words that we hear, can affect the physiology of the body, whether by hormonal release or by some other neurobiological mechanism.

In his introduction to Cousins's second book, *The Healing Heart*, so scrupulously scientific a clinician as Bernard Lown wrote about the "lethal power of words."[10] He told of a middle-aged woman who had been in relatively good health with "low grade congestive heart failure" at her regular visits to the clinic of Dr. Samuel Levine, a renowned Boston heart specialist. On one occasion, however, that noted physician announced to a group of students around the patient, "This woman has TS" and abruptly left.

> No sooner was Dr. Levine out of the door than Mrs. S's demeanor abruptly changed. She appeared anxious and frightened and was now breathing rapidly. . . . I found it astonishing that the lungs, which a few minutes earlier had been quite clear, now had moist crackles at the bases. . . . I questioned Mrs. S as to the reasons for her sudden upset. Her response what that Dr. Levine had said that she had TS, which she knew meant "terminal situation."

In fact TS stood for tricuspid-stenosis, only a chronic heart valve deformity. But the misunderstanding quickly led to the patient's worsening and "Later that same day she died from intractable heart failure. To this day, the recollection of this tragic happening causes me to tremble at the awesome power of the physician's word." As so often, Cousins phrases it remarkably well:

> Words, when used by the doctor, can be gate openers or gate slammers. They can open the way to recovery, or they can make a patient dependent, tremulous, fearful, resistant. The right words can potentiate a patient, mobilize the will to live, and provide a congenial environment for heroic response. The wrong words can produce despair. (p. 13)

10. Lown, B., quoted in N. Cousins, The healing heart, New York: Norton, 1983.

The therapeutic word is, after all, a reality, but it is a reality unfortunately, nowadays, heard mainly outside orthodox medical practice. Healing has many different sources. If movies can bring us to tears, or thrill us, and if we weep at some reading, sound, talk, the words of another, or music, can words change the direction of our perception? In connection with Cousins, Lown quotes Sydenham: "The arrival of a good clown exercises more beneficial influence upon the health of a town than twenty asses laden with drugs." Physicians should try to use more words in their practice, relying on suggestion, on words which can be taken in by the patient as much as the pills we prescribe. Words of persuasion and suggestion can address issues of personalistic origin, the illnesses which come from within. Physicians can influence the pain, suffering, and misery of illness, reserving drugs, diets, and surgery for the more "naturalistic" phenomena of disease.

Bourne suggested that the physician himself can be a vehicle for the placebo:

> In this broader sense the placebo is always indicated, as a necessary adjunct to specific drugs. We often assume that compassion and experience on the part of the physician are enough, and that the fears and hopes of patients will in effect take care of themselves. Everyday life provides abundant evidence, however, that personal relationships, especially in a setting of stress, can be far more difficult—even dangerous—than many of the intellectual judgements required for proper management of patients. . . . Honest straightforward communication can relieve anxiety. Perhaps more important, this sort of placebo may make fewer and less toxic drugs necessary to produce satisfactory relief of the patient's discomfort.[11]

Physicians respect mind-body relationships, but usually treat only the body. Again, we can ask if a story can make us weep, why can a story not also begin to engender "healing" of illness? Giving a placebo relieves complaints by modifying perceptions. When we give a placebo, we are simply giving a symbol, taking a shortcut. The placebo is only the first step, the beginning symbol of the healing process, for illness.

The Symbol of the Placebo

The placebo should be a symbol, a sacrament almost, for physician as well as for patient. It is not a magic ritual substituting for the process of clinical evaluation, but it does suggest changes in the patient-physician relationship focussing on illness as much as disease. The

11. Bourne, H. R., The placebo: A poorly understood and neglected therapeutic agent, *Rational Drug Therapy*, 5:1–5, 1971.

prescription may seal the therapeutic contract between doctor and patient.[12] During the dialogue of the history and physical the physician decides whether his patient needs an overt contract like a seal, or whether assurance that "You're in fine shape," the unrolling of a diagnostic approach, giving dietary instructions, or some other approach will suffice. The seal can be a pill or a procedure or sometimes only reassurance. Not everyone needs a pill; very few people at present need placebos.

Yet thinking about the placebo as sealing the therapeutic contract makes the transaction an explicit one. Some people need symbolic relief and placebos may be given only to establish trust. Giving a prescription like the old legal seal provides a ceremony which stops the transaction long enough to make everyone aware of what they are getting into. Heating up the sealing wax to put a ring into it underlined the seriousness of the contract. To write a prescription for a pill or a placebo should do the same. The patient must trust the doctor, but the doctor must also trust the patient. Prescribing a placebo should never be a substitute for time and energy but only the promise of dedication.

Contemplation of the power and the promise of the placebo could bridge the chasm between the naturalistic, rationalistic basis of our profession, and the personalistic, priestly, intuitive contribution that we physicians should still bring to medical practice and that many of us have rejected because of our training.

The Placebo as Part of the Healing System

For most patients getting a placebo should be only the first step in getting better, and only a small and tentative step at that, the beginning of a relationship between doctor and patient, which depends on talking, listening, and communicating as much as on looking and measuring. The doctor who gives a pill should take on an obligation to care for the patient, to be loyal to his needs. The patient also takes on an obligation, which I will not here discuss, to be an active partner in the therapeutic alliance.[13] The placebo given in an honest attempt to help, to a patient who expects something (and there are many), in an approach which says, "You and I don't know how or why my giving you this pill helps, but it will help," stands for the magical, mystical side of medicine. But it is more than that when given by a careful, caring physician who has not abandoned his patient and who will talk

12. Byck, R., Psychologic factors in drug administration, pp. 110–126, in *Clinical Pharmacology*, ed. K. Melman and H. Morelli, New York: Macmillan, 1978.

13. Gutheil, T. G., and Havens, L. L., The therapeutic alliance: Contemporary meanings and confusions, *Int. Rev. Psycho. Anal.* 6:467–79, 1979.

with him. We can have both science and intuition, if the placebo is given to seal the contract, by a doctor who will loyally serve his patient, and as Katz puts it, will not abandon him.[14]

Placebo or Active Drug?

Should a placebo be given for "real" disease to relieve pain when a more specific drug will change structural or functional origins of the pain? After all, the argument goes, if peptic ulcer pain or even angina can be relieved by symbolically evoking healing power or changing the cortical perception of the pain, why not use an agent which has no real side effects before anything stronger with other more "real" side effects? In an individual patient, as a matter of clinical judgment, I might feel that a placebo would prove effective, but as a matter of general policy, for now, I must still acclaim the active drug. Even if peptic ulcer pain is as readily relieved by a placebo as by biologically more active drugs such as H2 blockers, it makes current sense to use the active or logical drug. Healing is, after all, speeded up by cimetidine or ranitidine and this counts for something. Moreover the patient with an intractable ulcer is no longer a problem, a change I am happy to ascribe to the use of H2 blockers. As a general rule most physicians would feel uncomfortable giving a placebo instead of nitroglycerine to patients with angina pectoris, for example.

Yet the question persists, if 60 percent of ulcers heal on their own in controlled trials, why not rely on the meeting of physician and patient, awaiting outcome before using active drugs? Why not, in fact, use a placebo, if that is what milk or diet represent, in preference to logical pharmaceutical agents? Do we need to treat half the patients whose ulcer would disappear on scrutiny alone? Or hurry along the healing? The nitroglycerine patch over the heart to relieve or prevent angina has been widely acclaimed by physician and patient alike. Yet much evidence suggests that the effect has been only that of a placebo. Would any self-respecting cardiologist have put a patch of innocent tape over the heart in an honest attempt to relieve pain? What should we now think? More discussion is needed, but the current climate of opinion will not support the idea of placebo treatment for most diseases.

Indications for Placebo

There is a place for the placebo, but it is, after all, a small place. A placebo should be prescribed only after careful clinical evaluation, after explanation and reassurance and the launching of a diagnostic plan, if one seems necessary. There are people who need and benefit

14. Katz, J., *The silent world of doctor and patient*, New York: Free Press, 1984.

from this tangible sign of help. But the physician must give more than the prescription when he orders a placebo, he must give himself, or at least try, for the placebo stands as another kind of symbol, of all that the physician does that is not quantifiable, and that is what this book is all about.

A placebo can be used to try to wean the patient with addiction or habituation from his drugs; placebos can be given to the patient with pain from cancer before other drugs are used, but only if they give relief; and they should be used, with all the foregoing promises and understanding, in patients with pain of uncertain cause. Patients with chronic pain of uncertain cause may benefit the most. They want something for their pain, understandably enough, and it makes medical sense to try a placebo first before embarking on the use of more habituating agents.

There are also people, how many I do not know, to whom a placebo should be prescribed as a tangible symbol of healing from the first meeting. They may be hypochondriacs, people long accustomed to the behavioral benefit of a gift from the doctor. To take a broad stand against a placebo for such patients seems impractical, but a placebo is no substitute for an attempt at more. Many physicians, energetic and dedicated, have told how patients have asked for medication, even after a long discussion and examination. "What are you going to give me for this pain?" For such patients, magic and a gift, suggestion, have a place. Doctors need not feel guilty, as they so often do, in such circumstances. They need only remember that the romantic plays a part in medicine as much as the rational. It is as difficult for some patients to take an active role in their own treatment as it is for some doctors to let them.

The physician writes a prescription for his patient, saying that the pill may help. At the least, the pill simply focuses attention. Like any other icon or image, it concentrates the mind. Not everyone needs a pill as a placebo. In the past bloodletting, cupping, and other fancied therapeutic approaches, may have served the same symbolic function that X-rays and other diagnostic studies, and some therapeutic maneuvers, in part serve today. One other very practical virtue of the placebo is that while the patient is taking it, time is passing during which the natural tendency of acute disorders to improve lets the patient get better on his own, or gives the physician time to decide what to do. Giving a placebo may take the place of a sequence of diagnostic tests to reassure the patient and to make the physician feel that he is doing something. Of course giving an explanation and taking time to listen and to talk could be just as effective, but, as I have emphasized, for some explanation is not as comforting as a prescription.

Ritual plays a comforting role for most humans. The setting of the hospital or the doctor's office cannot be ignored any more than the temples of Aesculapius by the sea. The patient who journeys to a world-famous clinic or physician is as ready to be helped as the pilgrim who travels to a shrine, what Brody has called the "healing context." The site and circumstances of the meeting between physician and patient must play a role.

Brody comments:

> The placebo effect is most likely to occur when the following conditions are optimally met:
>
> 1) The patient is provided with an explanation for his illness which is consistent with his preexisting view of the world.
>
> 2) A group of individuals assuming socially sanctioned caring roles is available to provide emotional support for the patient.
>
> 3) The healing intervention leads to the patient's acquiring a sense of mastery and control over the illness.[15]

Some day, I hope, the placebo will prove unnecessary even as an icon, symbol of the physician's willingness to help. Let physicians only realize that on their own they are therapeutic, that by suggestion and persuasion, by words and little deeds, they can influence and comfort many patients and the placebo will serve ever less purpose. For patients, too, in that distant world, research and education will help us all to realize that within us there is the ability to relieve pain, to counteract depression and anxiety, to heal illness. Getting a pill will no longer be important to trigger such responses. Now the placebo serves as a convenient focus for the physician, reminding him that he is treating a human being just as it tells the patient that his doctor is more than a vending machine of techniques or a technician supplying pills. But once physicians and patients are free of thinking that only technology and pills can help, then patient and physician alike may rely much more on the healing alliance in which illness is comforted. Dialogue, communication, all the kinds of community that we have been talking about, will prove as powerful. But only for illness.

We can have it both ways, science and intuition, reason and romanticism. Both-and, not either-or. There is room for both in medicine and the dichotomies I have set up for discussion turn out to be only parts of a whole. For the physician, there should be no split between natural sciences and "the sciences of the spirit" of the German idealists. Not all patients are the same, some require more art and some more science. Science and intuition are not mutually exclusive, certainly not in the care of people. The benefits of empathy and commu-

15. Brody. H., *Placebos and the philosophy of medicine*, Chicago: University of Chicago Press, 1980.

nication may be as great, sometimes, as pills and potions, but when they are not, placebos can help and physicians need not feel guilty that they turn to the magical side of their work.

I have tried to make it clear that I am convinced that diseases, the structurally determined changes in the body, need the services of a physician. There are, alas, few proven miracles, and the slow, steady progress of scientific medicine, along with improvement in the environment and the enormous expansion of public health services and preventive medicine, have been responsible—it is my faith—for the improved state of health in the Western world. Yet these reflections suggest that the Western medical system has currently done away with all other forms of healing. The past decade has seen the expansion of alternative medicine, and much of this is surely to the good. Indeed there are many signs within the medical profession that concerned physicians have for some years been using alternative principles of healing. It has been my purpose also to suggest that illness, whether the response to pressure or the stress of having an organic structural disease, can be treated, as it has been for so long in the past, by other forms of caring people and professionals. But those responses are a testimony to our common humanity, to the wonder that one person can help another.

The placebo gives a promise of what medical practice can become even in an era of technology. The physician stands between the patient and the power of modern technology. The old priests of Apollo propitiated the gods; the modern physician controls the mysterious forces of science for the human patients he or she serves. The placebo tells us that cure and care depend on science and on art, but that sometimes poetry may offer the patient as much as physics, that the physician should treat despair along with disease. The placebo as gift and promise from one person to another stands against the icon, symbol of technology and power. In an era of imaging, the placebo reminds us that patients are more than their icons, that patients are people. The placebo stands for office practice, reminding us of the differences between complaints which are 80 percent illness and diseases which is what the hospitals are all about. To generate an image you need machinery, computers, the power of the hospital, where the white coat is an appropriate symbol. To give a placebo the doctor needs only hands and a mind. The icon enshrines disease at a distance, sterile without emotion, serene and dispassionate but above all rational. The placebo is given one to another, here and now, in a mystery which is at the same time irrational and in the romantic tradition. The symbol of the icon is the eye. The placebo needs the ear. The icon may give us truth and show us disease, but the placebo brings comfort to the person.

The placebo has no power, only a promise.

Index

Acupuncture: cultural context of, 162–63; evaluating effectiveness of for pain, 175–77; explanations of, 101, 105, 164

Aesculapian medicine, 173

Alternative medicine: characteristics of, 147–48; constituency for, 90, 147–48, 182, 184–85, 243–44, 253; Cousins case, 107–13; definition of, 146–47; evaluating effects of, 6–7, 146, 167–69; weaknesses of, 181–82. *See also* Acupuncture

Angina pectoris, 250; placebo effects of drugs in, 13, 86, 87; placebo effects of mammary artery ligation for, 42, 44

Ankylosing spondylitis, 108

Anorexia nervosa, cultural context of, 167

Antibiotics, 135–36, 139

Anxiety, 52; effects of on placebo responses, 92, 93, 96; prescribing for, 24

Art of Ministering to the Sick, The (Cabot and Dicks), 120–21

Aspirin, 7–8

Attention: in clinical trials, 13; costs of, 183; in Crohn's disease, 16–17; in esophageal spasm, 45; Hawthorne effect, 14; healing power of, 182, 184; placebo as focusing device for, 219, 222, 251; as therapy, 17. *See also* Care; Care *vs.* cure

Attitudes. *See* Belief; Intent

Autonomy: and control of placebo, 112–13; disadvantages of for patients, 113–

16; effects of illness on, 125–26, 127; effects of on physicians' role, 31; as goal of treatment, 111–12; limiting, 144, 244; priority of, 127; and transference, 220

Behavioral mechanisms. *See* Conditioned responses

Behavioral therapy, 216–17

Belief: effects of on physician as healer, 34–35; in holistic medicine, 181; and intent in placebo transaction, 24, 26–27; in medicine *vs.* healing, 28; placebo effects of, 44. *See also* Intent

Biasing, in pain perception, 102

Biomedical model, and medical anthropology, 170–71

Biopsychosocial medical model, 59–61

Blood sugar, 82–83

Bouginage, as placebo, 45

Bowel disease, 56, 59

Brain, *vs.* mind, 52–55

Buchanan, Allen, 127–28

Cabot, Hugh, 121

Cabot, Richard, 118–22

Cabot, Ted, 121–22

Cancers: placebo effects in, 77–78, 90; spontaneous remission *vs.* placebo effects in, 78–80

Care: giving drugs as symbol of, 239; overuse of technology in, 3–4. *See also* Attention

255